Adult Medicine

MODERN PRACTICAL NURSING SERIES

This important new nursing series, designed specifically for the State Enrolled Nurse and Auxiliary Nurse is published as a 'parent' book covering the basic nursing skills entitled AN OUTLINE OF BASIC NURSING CARE, and a number of smaller handbooks covering the individual specialities as the nurse is moved from one discipline to another.

AN OUTLINE OF BASIC NURSING CARE: This aims to help the nurse learn the general basic nursing skills and also how to apply them, and stimulate thought about nursing in different hospital situations.

THE SPECIALITY BOOKS: Having mastered the basic nursing skills the pupil nurse will find herself attached to the nursing staff in any ward in the hospital. Although she is expected to play a part in this specialised ward team she may have had only a brief glimpse of the subject in her earlier training. It is for this stage in her career that this series of books is designed. The subjects covered include: Paediatric Orthopaedics, Theatre Routine, Paediatric Surgery, Dermatology, Urology, Adult Medicine, Geriatrics, Ear Nose and Throat, Mental Deficiency, Ophthalmology, Adult Orthopaedics, Plastic Surgery and Burns Treatment, Psychiatry, Obstetrics, and Adult Surgery. All these are written by expert authors usually consisting of a doctor and sister tutor actively engaged in the work about which they have written and in touch with modern nursing trends.

These books are extensively illustrated and easy to use. As paperbacks they are inexpensive and it is hoped therefore that the nurse will have available a set of modern practical books which will help her in her ward work.

9 Modern Practical Nursing Series

Adult Medicine

R.D. Barr, MB, ChB, MRCP.
Registrar; Medical Department, Glasgow Royal Infirmary.

E.H.R. Laird, RGN, SCM, HV.
Sister Tutor, Glasgow Royal Infirmary School of Nursing.

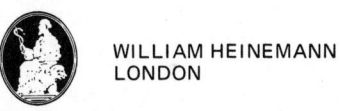

WILLIAM HEINEMANN MEDICAL BOOKS
LONDON

First Published 1971
© E.H.R. Laird and R.D. Barr 1971
ISBN 0 433 19050 7
Printed in Great Britain by
Redwood Press Limited
Trowbridge & London

CONTENTS

Chapter		Page
	Introduction	
	Section I	1
1	Diseases of the Alimentary System	3
2	Diseases of the Respiratory System	15
3	Diseases of the Blood and Blood-Forming Organs	25
4	Diseases of the Locomotor System	34
5	Diseases of the Pituitary	36
6	Diseases of the Thyroid	38
7	Diseases of the Adrenals	41
8	Diseases of the Pancreas	44
9	Diseases of the Kidneys	48
10	Diseases of the Heart and Blood Vessels	53
11	Diseases of the Nervous System	65
	Section II	71
	Patient Care	73
	General Nursing Duties	75
	Nursing Care in Congestive Cardiac Failure	86
	Nursing Care in Left Ventricular Failure	88
	Nursing Care in Myocardial Infarction	88
	Nursing Care in Deep Vein Thrombosis	90
	Nursing Care in Pulmonary Embolism	91
	Nursing Care of the Hypertensive Patient	91
	Nursing Care Following Cerebro-Vascular Accident	92
	Nursing Care in Diabetes Mellitus	94
	Nursing Care in Thyrotoxicosis	98

Chapter	Page
Nursing Care for the Patient with Jaundice	99
Nursing Care in Respiratory Infection	99
Nursing Care for Patient with Anaemia	100
Nursing Care in Haematemesis and Melaena	101
Nursing Care for Patients with Ulcerative Colitis	102
Nursing Care of the Epileptic Patient	103
Nursing Care in Acute Poisoning	103

Section III

Special Diagnostic Procedures	107
1. Sternal Marrow Puncture	109
2. Iliac Crest Biopsy	109
3. Fibroscopy	112
4. Crosby Capsule	113
5. Renal Biopsy	114
6. Liver Biopsy	116
7. Histamine Test Meal	117
8. Aspiration of the Peritoneal Cavity	119
9. Aspiration of the Pleural Cavity	120
10. Proctoscopy, Sigmoidoscopy, Rectal Biopsy	122
11. Lumbar Puncture	122
12. Passing Tubes	124
	126
Glossary of Terms	
Index	127
Pages for Notes	131

INTRODUCTION

The book is in three sections principally because it was evident there would be repetition of procedures and nursing care if the nursing section was integrated into the medical section.

The three sections are allied to each other in content.

Section I — Medical — principal conditions affecting each system of the body.

Section II — Nursing Care and Procedures — covering the most frequently occuring conditions found in the acute medical ward.

Section III — Special Diagnostic Procedures.

It must at the outset be appreciated that this text is not intended to be comprehensive, many topics, for example, carcinoma of the bowel, being covered entirely or more fully by other texts in the series.

R.D.B.

The Nursing Section of this book is intended to give information which will improve knowledge and practical nursing skills. It is hoped this will give greater understanding and satisfaction in medical nursing experience.

E.L.

Section I

Only the most important diseases are included and discussed, their importance being determined by the frequency with which a nurse will encounter them, and/or their value in highlighting certain basic principles. An attempt is made to lay emphasis on those aspects of patient management in which the nurse is particularly involved. The individual diseases will be discussed systematically and as far as possible according to the following scheme.

Disease
1) Cause
2) Methods of diagnosis
   a) Symptoms
   b) Physical signs
   c) Investigations
3) Treatment
   a) Specific
   b) Supportive
4) Prognosis

In many diseases, for example, disseminated sclerosis, the cause is not known, and where this is the case it is so stated, but in other conditions the cause is well established, e.g., the virus producing shingles.

Diagnosis is the process of identification of a disease. Symptoms are the complaints which the patient makes to the doctor spontaneously and in response to appropriate questions, for example, pain in the arm. Physical signs which may be normal or abnormal, are items of information elicited by the doctor on clinical examination of the patient, for example, counting the pulse rate. Investigations are tests performed by the nursing, medical and laboratory staff which are designed to confirm the clinical diagnosis based on the symptoms and physical signs, for example, testing a sample of urine for protein in a patient with suspected kidney disease.

For the majority of diseases there is no specific cure, but in most instances there are generally accepted principles by which treatment is governed, for example, dietary restriction in diabetes mellitus.

However for some diseases there are specific cures, for example, Vitamin C for scurvy. Supportive treatment, in which the nurse commonly plays a major role, often offers the patient considerable relief from his distress and contributes to his recovery, for example, tepid sponging and administration of a liberal fluid intake in a patient with pneumonia.

Prognosis is an assessment of the eventual outcome of a disease.

1
Diseases of the Alimentary System

The Mouth

Cold Sores
The result of a virus infection, these are groups of small painful blisters usually on and around the lips. They commonly occur as an isolated finding, but may be seen in association with pneumonia and meningitis. There is no cure and they tend to recur although local applications such as Glycerine may relieve the discomfort.

Thrush
A yeast infection, this appears as small white areas usually inside the mouth. It tends to occur in very ill patients, especially those who may be diabetic or suffering from cancer or who have been receiving certain antibiotics. Cure usually results from local application of Gentian violet or Nystatin.

Sore Tongue
A feature of many conditions, the most common of which is anaemia, classically pernicious anaemia, the tongue is often red, smooth, shiny and painful and may even be swollen. Frequently there is improvement or cure on appropriately treating the underlying disease.

The Oesophagus

Cancer
Cause unknown. Usually encountered in old men. The patient nearly always complains of progressive difficulty in swallowing, first of solids and later of liquids, often associated with loss of weight, which may be striking. X-ray examination of the oesophagus (Barium swallow) usually reveals where the tumour is obstructing the passage of food stuffs. The surgeon may examine the oesophagus through an oesophagoscope and visualise the growth directly. A combination of surgical removal of the tumour and radiotherapy offers the only slim hope of cure, for the disease is commonly fatal.

If the former is not technically possible, various palliative

Diseases of the Alimentary System

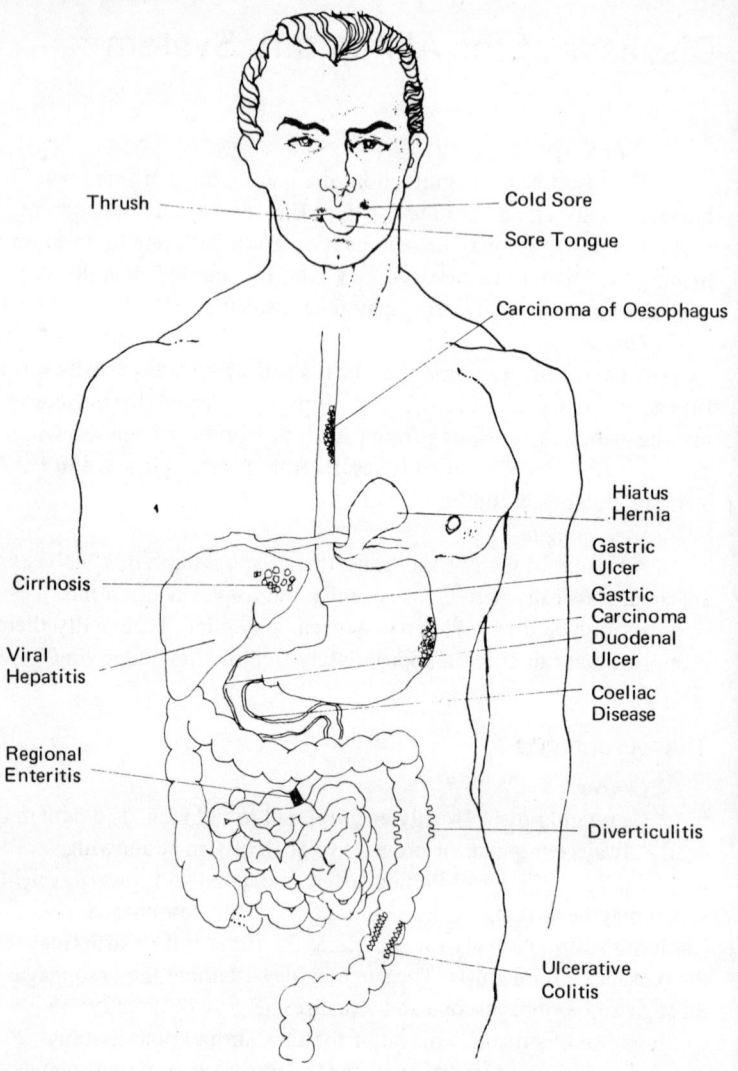

procedures may allow the patient to swallow, so making more comfortable the short period of time which may elapse before death.

Heart-burn

This is a burning sensation experienced in the centre of the chest and usually reflects inflammation in the oesophagus which may be due to acid flowing into it from the stomach. Antacid therapy will often relieve the discomfort and the patient should be encouraged to avoid those factors which may provoke the symptom, for example, over-eating.

The Stomach

Hiatus Hernia

A part of the stomach becomes displaced through the opening in the diaphragm by which the oesophagus normally enters the abdomen and joins the stomach. Hence the affected part of the stomach comes to lie in the chest and so gastric acid more easily enters the oesophagus giving rise to heart burn. Conditions which predispose to the development of this abnormality include obesity, pregnancy and chronic constipation in all of which the pressure inside the abdomen is increased and tends to force part of the stomach into the chest. X-ray examination (Barium meal) commonly reveals the portion of stomach in its abnormal position. Conservative measures such as dietary restriction, relief of constipation, avoidance of stooping and lying flat (which facilitates the entry of gastric acid into the oesophagus), taking antacid therapy, and advising the patient to sleep propped up will usually result in notable improvement. Only infrequently is it necessary to resort to operation and return the displaced stomach to the abdomen.

Gastric ulcer

Although seen less frequently than duodenal ulcer this is by no means an uncommon condition. It is probably due to an imbalance between the amount of acid produced by the stomach and the resistance of the stomach wall to the action of the acid, so that the wall becomes damaged by the acid and an ulcer forms. Pain is the most prominent symptom. It is experienced, by most patients, in the upper abdomen and usually occurs within one hour of eating a meal. Characteristically appetite is depressed, vomiting often results in relief of discomfort, and weight loss may be noted. Sometimes complications occur, the two common events being bleeding and perforation. In the former situation the patient may vomit blood, while in the latter he usually develops peritonitis as a result of the contents of the stomach escaping through a hole in the ulcer and soiling the peritoneal cavity. Examination of a patient with a gastric ulcer often reveals tenderness at the site of his pain. The presence of the ulcer may be confirmed by X-ray examination (Barium meal) and by directly visualising the lesion through a gastroscope passed into the stomach. The majority of gastric ulcers heal on conservative treatment. Patients should be advised to rest, to stop smoking, and to take antacids for relief of pain. Healing is promoted by certain drugs made from extracts of the liquorice plant. Gastric ulcers tend to recur and affected patients may eventually require to undergo surgery. Surgical intervention is of course more frequently necessary for the management of bleeding and perforation.

Cancer

As with cancer of the oesophagus this all too common tumour is usually encountered in older subjects. Although the cause is quite unknown it is significantly more common in patients with pernicious anaemia. Loss of appetite and profound weight loss are usual and pain and vomiting similar to that of gastric ulcer may occur. Bleeding into the stomach may result but perforation is uncommon. The patient often appears pale and emaciated and not infrequently the tumour may be palpable and even visible in the upper abdomen. The clinical diagnosis may be confirmed by the same techniques as those applied in the demonstration of a gastric ulcer. Surgical removal of the tumour offers the only possibility of cure. Unfortunately in many instances this is technically impossible and even in those patients whose tumours are apparently excised the chances of long term survival are remote, since tiny portions of tumour are often missed by even the most careful of surgeons and by the time patients are submitted to operation unrecognised spread of the tumour may already have occurred. Like patients with cancer of the oesophagus these patients require skilled nursing care with due consideration being paid in particular to achieving relief of pain by the administration of appropriate analgesics and the provision of such nutrition as the patient feels able to tolerate.

The Small Bowel

Duodenal Ulcer

A very common condition, there is a greater likelihood of an individual developing such an ulcer if other members of his family are known to have the disease. Again, although the cause is not known with certainty, the great majority of patients who have duodenal ulcers have stomachs which produce more than normal amounts of acid. Upper abdominal pain is usually experienced before meals and one to two hours or even longer after meals and frequently is responsible for waking the patient at night. Characteristically pain is relieved by taking food or antacids, appetite is retained, vomiting is uncommon, and body weight is either unchanged or increased as a result of drinking large quantities of milk to obtain relief from pain. As in cases of gastric ulcer the patient may experience intermittent periods of weeks or months with freedom from symptoms. Bleeding is a common complication and is manifest in a large number of instances as vomiting of blood (haematemesis) and the passage of dark or frankly black stools (melaena).

Perforation of a duodenal ulcer is a cause of many hospital admissions. This emergency situation is classically attended by sudden onset of severe generalised abdominal pain, the patient rapidly developing peritonitis. A further, rather less common, but by no means rare complication is that of pyloric stenosis, in which there is a narrowing of that part of the stomach which communicates with the duodenum, resulting from shrinkage of the scarring which accompanies the ulcer. This produces hold-up in the passage of partially digested food onwards from the stomach which therefore becomes greatly enlarged and the patient has to vomit massive amounts of material to obtain relief from abdominal distension. Localised upper abdominal tenderness is a notable feature of many cases of duodenal ulcer and is much more marked and widespread following perforation. The patient who has suffered a large haemorrhage almost invariably appears shocked with pallor, a rapid thready pulse, and low blood pressure, while pyloric stenosis is characteristically accompanied by an audible splash in the dilated stomach when the patient's abdomen is shaken. Barium meal examination may demonstrate the presence of the ulcer or the resulting scarring or both and is useful in confirming the complication of pyloric stenosis.

The conservative management of a patient with a duodenal ulcer consists of rest, if possible in bed, the avoidance of alcohol and food stuffs such as spices if these precipitate abdominal pain, the use of antacid therapy, and the taking of regular frequent small meals. However, in many patients, this regime fails to relieve the symptoms. Certain liquorice extracts may provide a solution to the problem of healing established ulcers but at present a significant proportion of patients suffering from an uncomplicated duodenal ulcer eventually require surgical intervention. The majority of episodes of bleeding resulting from duodenal ulceration halt spontaneously and so with careful monitoring of pulse and blood pressure and the testing of stools and aspirated gastric juice for blood, all designed to assess the degree of bleeding, combined with the transfusion of blood as required to make up the loss the patient usually avoids an operation at this stage. Perforation and pyloric stenosis however are virtually certain indications for surgical management.

Coeliac disease

One of the commonest of the diseases leading to the 'malabsorption syndrome' this appears to be due to an acquired sensitivity to gluten, a protein fraction of wheat, leading to the development of an anatomically and functionally abnormal lining of the small bowel, that part of the gut which plays the most important role in absorption of digested food stuffs. With the failure to absorb ingested material the patient characteristically complains of passing pale, bulky and offensive stools which tend to float unduly on water. These features are largely related to the high quantity of fat in such faeces. Consequent on the failure of absorption, affected patients almost invariably lose weight and readily become anaemic. A striking feature on examination of some patients is distension of the abdomen, especially in children. Patients with this disease require extensive investigation both to establish the diagnosis and to determine the nature and degree of the deficiencies which have resulted from malabsorption. X-ray examination (Barium follow through) may reveal an abnormal appearance of the small bowel, a tiny portion of the lining of which may be obtained via a Crosby capsule and subsequently submitted to microscopic examination. Collection of stools over a period of at least four days allows calculation of their content of fat, while a variety of other less specific tests will allow estimation of the various deficiencies of iron, protein and vitamins which may have occurred. Treatment consists essentially of withdrawal of gluten from the diet and replacement of the various materials which the patient has come to lack as a result of diminished ability to absorb them. Many patients return to normality on this regime.

Regional Enteritis

An inflammatory disease, the cause of which remains quite unknown, this may affect any part of the gut from the oesophagus to the anus, though it is usually localised to or predominantly affects the small bowel. The bowel is usually involved in patches rather than continuously. Abdominal pain and diarrhoea are the main symptoms and they may be accompanied by a fever. Weight loss is not uncommon. The characteristic complication of regional enteritis is the formation of abnormal connections between adjacent loops of small bowel which have become matted together as a result of the disease. Patients are often anaemic and in a notable proportion a tender mass may be felt in the abdomen. This is usually composed of loops of bowel which have been affected by the inflammatory process. Further confirmation of the diagnosis may be obtained from X-ray examination of the small bowel. No uniformly successful treatment is available but improvement has been achieved with steroid therapy and Salazopyrin, a drug which has proved useful in the management of ulcerative colitis. Selected patients may benefit from specialised surgical management, especially those who develop complications. The eventual outcome for the individual patient is almost impossible to assess at the onset of his illness. Some apparently become cured, but many become progressively more ill and after several years may die as a result of the disease.

The Large Bowel

Diverticulitis

The complication arising in a small minority of elderly patients with the benign condition of diverticulosis, this disease is basically an inflammation of some of the small pouches which are present in the large bowel in these patients. The main and frequently the only symptom is that of lower abdominal pain. Occasionally one of the inflamed pouches bursts and peritonitis may result. Other complications are far less common. Careful palpation of the abdomen may allow the doctor to feel a tender lower abdominal mass which represents the inflamed bowel. Treatment is essentially conservative, at least in the first instance. It is important to prevent constipation and the diet is therefore adjusted accordingly. Resort to operation may sometimes have to be made, particularly if peritonitis occurs. Since this disease occurs almost invariably in elderly people, it rarely results in a shortening of their life expectancy.

Ulcerative colitis

Largely affecting younger subjects this condition has long perplexed the physician and surgeon alike. Although, by no means firmly established or uniformly accepted, the present popular theory is that the disease results from the patient developing intolerance and a reaction to his own bowel as if it were foreign material. This reaction produces a marked inflammation in the wall of the large bowel which may in severe cases be affected along its entire length. Usually the disease begins in the last section of the bowel, the rectum and lower colon, and may remain localised or spread to affect other areas of the gut. The initial symptoms may be mild or drastically severe and may begin slowly or with dramatic suddeness. In the characteristic severe case the patient's major complaint is most frequently of profuse watery diarrhoea with the passage of more than 20 stools per day accompanied by fresh blood, mucus and pus per rectum. This is associated with loss of appetite, abdominal pain relieved by defaecation, rapid loss of weight and the feeling that even after defaecation the rectum is not empty. Many patients however experience much milder symptoms.

Complications are the hallmark of this disease. The most important are haemorrhage from the inflamed bowel; dilatation and perforation of the bowel leading to peritonitis; the establishment of abnormal communications between sections of bowel as in regional enteritis; the formation of strictures in the bowel, as a result of scarring, leading to intestinal obstruction; and the development of cancer in the affected section of bowel. Very ill patients may be in shock and may demonstrate the signs of peritonitis, while the mildly affected patient may only reveal slight lower abdominal tenderness. X-ray examination of the bowel (Barium enema) usually demonstrates an abnormal appearance if the disease has extended beyond the rectum and lower colon. Direct examination of these areas through a sigmoidoscope will allow any affected part to be visualised and a tiny fragment of the bowel wall may be removed and examined under a microscope. Management of the severely ill patient with ulcerative colitis demands the highest skill from all medical and nursing staff involved, since many patients have died in this phase of the illness.

There are two main forms of medical treatment, and these involve the use of steroid drugs which may be given by mouth, by injection, or by enema, and Salazopyrin, which is given by mouth. Supportive measures are all important and these include maintenance of water, salt and calorie balance and attendance to pressure areas. Careful watch must be kept continuously for evidence of deterioration in the patients condition such as a rise in temperature or pulse rate, a fall in blood pressure, or the appearance of abdominal distension. Less severely affected patients of course require only a modification of the regime. Should the patient fail to respond to medical management or should complications arise the advice and help of an experienced surgeon should be sought. The progress of the disease is usually one of remission and relapse and while some patients with mild symptoms can be managed conservatively, a high proportion will eventually require surgical operation.

The Liver

Viral Hepatitis

The commoner form of this disease, infectious hepatitis, is usually contracted by the affected patient consuming food or water which has been contaminated by infected faeces, while the other form of the disease, serum hepatitis is usually contracted by the affected patient receiving an injection with materials or instruments which have been in contact with infected blood. The incubation period for the latter disease form is longer than that for the former but otherwise the two forms are very similar.

Prominent symptoms are marked loss of appetite, nausea, loss of desire to smoke, upper abdominal discomfort, pale stools, dark urine, generalised itch and the development of jaundice. Many patients do not become jaundiced and in these it may be difficult to make the diagnosis. Characteristically the liver is enlarged and tender and jaundice is evident. Simple inspection of the stools may confirm that they are pale while chemical testing of the urine may reveal the presence of bile and excess urobilinogen. Numerous blood tests are performed to look for evidence of upset in the liver function. In the uncomplicated case the management is simple and straight forward. The patient should be confined to bed till he begins to feel improved and he should be given a bland diet with a high content of carbohydrate. In the great majority of instances complete recovery occurs, but occasional patients suffer a severe form of the disease particularly with serum hepatitis and develop progressive jaundice, a bleeding tendency, confusion, convulsions and deepening coma with eventual death. There are virtually no measures which can be taken to remedy such situations. This disease draws attention to the necessity for good personal hygiene, for proper sterilisation of equipment and for adequate screening of blood donors so that no patient who has ever had jaundice is allowed to give blood.

Cirrhosis

While in a number of cases the cause of this disorder is well known, such as chronic alcoholism or hepatitis, in a high percentage of patients no underlying disease is apparent. The established condition is basically one in which the liver, probably in response to damage, often unrecognised, initially enlarges, becomes scarred and thereafter frequently progressively shrinks. In a small number of patients there may be no relevant symptoms and the diagnosis is suspected only after the incidental discovery of an enlarged liver, or some other feature of chronic liver disease, at physical examination. The remaining patients may complain of loss of appetite, undue tiredness and swelling of the legs and abdomen or more dramatically of symptoms related to bleeding into the gut, or the rapid onset of jaundice with drowsiness and confusion. Patients with the full blown clinical disorder will have jaundice, oedema of the legs, enlargement of the liver and spleen and abdominal distension due largely to the accumulation of free fluid (ascites). When there are no symptoms the liver function is usually well maintained but deterioration may occur at any time and may be produced by infections, drugs and anaesthetics among a variety of influences. Bleeding into the gut may arise from veins in the oesophagus which have become distended due to increased back pressure resulting from the diseased liver causing obstruction of the portal vein into which these smaller veins empty. Should liver function become sufficiently impaired toxic effects on the brain may develop resulting in confusion, tremors and even convulsions and death. If the diagnosis is suspected the urine should be tested for bile and excess urobilinogen, the stool for occult blood and the blood, by a variety of tests, to demonstrate defective liver function. A barium swallow examination may reveal the presence of the enlarged oesophageal veins while a biopsy of the liver itself often confirms the nature of the disease. Once the damage to the liver has become established, the patient cannot be cured but further damage may be largely avoided by such measures as abstaining from alcohol.

Those patients who have no symptoms, in general require no treatment but should be encouraged to take a diet low in salt and rich in protein and vitamins. When the liver shows signs of failing, dietary restriction of protein should be advised for at this stage the liver cannot properly utilize protein. Regular bowel movements are essential and an unabsorbed antibiotic such as Neomycin may have to be given to prevent the normal bacteria in the bowel from producing toxic materials which when absorbed cannot be dealt with by the unhealthy liver. Ascites and oedema of the legs may be relieved by the use of diuretics. The occurrence of gastro-intestinal bleeding in cirrhotic patients is often a situation of grave emergency and requires considerable skill and co-operation of medical and nursing personnel in the management of this life threatening complication. In addition to the manoeuvres described for the control of gastro-intestinal haemorrhage from peptic ulcers, cirrhotic patients in this dilemma may require injections of Pitressin to reduce the rate of bleeding or the passage of a Sengstaken tube to compress the oesophageal veins. Some patients may have to undergo surgery in an attempt to reduce the pressure in these dilated vessels and so reduce the risk of further bleeding, but this frequently results in further deterioration of liver function.

No shortening of the life expectancy occurs in those patients whose liver function does not progressively deteriorate or in whom no complications arise. As with all other patients with liver disease great care must be taken in drug administration since a considerable number of drugs may cause liver damage. When signs of confusion appear or when haemorrhage occurs the outlook is much less hopeful and although with careful management such patients may be tided over one or more of these events, generally the disease follows a downhill course with eventual death in coma or from uncontrollable haemorrhage.

2
Diseases of the Respiratory System

The Bronchi

Acute Bronchitis

When affecting previously healthy individuals this is commonly caused by a virus, often one of the influenza viruses, while patients who have established disease, especially a chronic respiratory disease, may suffer acute bacterial bronchitis. In any patient an acute non-infective bronchitis may result from inhaling toxic gases such as chlorine. The usual symptoms in the infective cases are initially those of a influenza-like illness with malaise, headache, generalised aches and pains, shivering and sweating being followed by a cough which soon becomes productive of mucopurulent sputum and may be accompanied by retrosternal pain. Examination usually reveals the patient to be febrile with only a few crepitations to be heard on listening over the chest. Frank pneumonia may supervene and less commonly collapse of a part of a lung may occur as a result of obstruction of a bronchus by secretions. In the absence of these complications the chest X-ray will be normal. Culture of the sputum is essential to investigate the possibility of a bacterial infection. If this is confirmed an appropriate antibiotic, usually one of the penicillins or tetracyclines should be given. For the standard case of acute viral bronchitis only supportive measures are required including bed rest, soluble aspirin and a cough suppressant such as codeine if the cough is irritating and non productive. The disease is always self limiting in previous healthy individuals.

Chronic Bronchitis and Emphysema.

These two entities are frequently associated, emphysema apparently resulting from long standing bronchitis. In emphysema, the lung substance, instead of being of a spongy consistency is represented by large sacs of air which in terms of respiration are poorly functioning. Cigarette smoking and atmospheric pollution are the main factors involved in the production of chronic bronchitis which is characterised by a persistent cough normally accompanied by mucoid or mucopurulent sputum. The sputum is particularly likely to become purulent during an episode of acute bacterial bronchitis to which these patients are especially susceptible. As the disease advances and progressive lung distortion occurs, increasing breathlessness becomes evident. Complications are a notable occurrence and may take the form of pneumonia during the course of an acute infection, spontaneous pneumothorax when an emphysematous air sac bursts or congestive cardiac failure when the damaged lungs provide too great a resistance to the flow of blood into them from the right side of the heart. Numerous patients have little or no abnormality on examination while others appear breathless and even exhibit wheezing particularly when suffering from an acute respiratory infection. In severely affected patients cyanosis may be present while in others, features of the complications may be noted. Characteristically the patient with long standing disease has a barrel shaped chest with poor respiratory movements and may or may not have crepitations consistent with excessive bronchial secretions. It is important to culture the sputum to determine the nature of the infecting organism and its sensitivity to antibiotics. Chest X-rays may be helpful but are often difficult to interpret in this situation

A variety of tests of respiratory function have been designed to assess the nature and severity of the patients disability and when performed on successive occasions may give a good estimate of progress or deterioration. All attempts should be made to encourage such patients to give up smoking and to avoid as far as possible exposure to atmospheric pollution. Emphysema is irreversible so treatment is directed towards control of the acute episodes of bronchitis with appropriate antibiotics. Bronchodilators such as Ephedrine may be useful in those patients in whom episodes of acute bronchitis are complicated by wheezing.

Sedatives and related drugs should be avoided in the great majority of these patients since they may so depress breathing that the patient enters a phase of respiratory failure. Another important point in management is the administration of oxygen to severely affected individuals. Most of these patients can tolerate only small amounts of oxygen and to exceed these again runs the risk of depressing respiration. Many patients live a normal life-span but most have a limited exercise tolerance as a result of their disease. A notable number of patients progressively deteriorate and die in late middle age or even earlier of respiratory or congestive cardiac failure.

Asthma.

Essentially a disorder in which the bronchi become narrowed as a result of constriction, usually in large part reversible, this is a disease often attributed to allergy. The patient may be allergic to a variety of external agents such as house dust which produce asthma when inhaled, or less commonly ingested foodstuffs or drugs. Other patients appear to develop an allergic response to chest infections which then become complicated by asthma. Typically asthmatic episodes occur at spasmodic intervals, the patient being essentially normal between attacks. Wheezing is the most prominent symptom, the patient taking a long time to exhale. This usually settles spontaneously within a few hours but may persist even for several days. The condition then being termed status asthmaticus. The chest is usually over-inflated during an attack reflecting the obstruction to expiration. On listening to the chest the classical high pitched expiratory wheeze is heard. Crepitations consistent with chest infection may also be audible.

Investigations are usually unnecessary and largely unhelpful in the diagnosis of bronchial asthma but the identification of the various agents to which the individual patient is allergic is a useful contribution and is usually accompanied by the technique of skin testing. Patients in whom this is successful may then be able to take suitable precautions to avoid undue exposure to these substances, while occasional fortunate patients may be at least temporarily desensitised by a series of injections of the offending agent in increasing strength. For the acute attack therapy may be started with subcutaneous Adrenaline. If this is ineffective intravenous Aminophylline will be required and should this too fail the administration of steroids often by continuous intravenous infusion will often prove necessary.

All personnel dealing with a patient suffering from an acute attack should be calm and confident and should reassure the patients, since this policy contributes significantly to the control of the attack. If chest infection is playing a part in the disease it should be appropriately treated. Many of the patients who develop asthma in childhood experience spontaneous cessation of attacks in early adult life. Persistent attacks of asthma from any cause may produce pulmonary emphysema.

Bronchiectasis.

Resulting from pulmonary infections, this is a chronic irreversible disorder involving dilation and destruction of the bronchial walls. It may become apparent many years after an episode of measles or whooping cough pneumonia in childhood or occur during the course of recurrent respiratory track infections. Cough is usually persistent and productive of very large volumes of purulent sputum often accompanied by haemoptysis although occasional patients produce very little sputum. Complicating episodes of frank pneumonia are common and are the usual mode of death. Other complications are encountered much less frequently. Severely affected patients are anaemic and wasted while the great majority have easily audible crepitations over the diseased areas of lung. Clubbing of the digits is a characteristic finding and features of pneumonia may be present. Culture of the sputum is essential to determine in particular the antibiotic sensitivity of the organisms present. Standard Chest X-rays may reveal a honeycomb or cystic appearance corresponding to the damaged parts of the lung. A radio-opaque absorbable dye may be introduced into the bronchi by means of which subsequent X-ray examination may demonstrate the distorted bronchial tree. This examination should be performed on separate occasions for each lung. A few patients who can be shown to have the disease strictly localised to one or two parts of a lung may be suitable candidates for surgical excision of these involved areas. However, most patients with bronchiectasis have more extensive disease and require to be managed conservatively. Such management should consist of vigorous physiotherapy with assisted coughing, postural drainage of the affected lung and deep breathing exercises. These should be performed early in the day and repeated as often as necessary. It is imperative that this regime be adhered to regularly on a daily basis. Episodes of pneumonia naturally require appropriate antibiotic therapy, while many patients who continuously produce large volumes of sputum will benefit from the administration of long-term broad spectrum antibiotics such as Tetracycline. The most severely affected patients will live only a few years before eventually succumbing to one of the many attacks of pneumonia to which they are particularly susceptible. Others who are minimally inconvenienced by their disease may enjoy a normal life expectancy.

The Lungs

Lobar Pneumonia.

Now seen less commonly in British practice, this is characteristically a disease of young adults. It is due to an acute infection of one or infrequently two lobes of a lung by the bacterium pneumococcus. The onset of the illness is classically abrupt with rigors, chest pain, and cough productive of rusty, blood stained sputum. Fever, dehydration and often herpes lesions on the lips are notable features. Examination of the chest usually reveals signs of consolidation of one of the lung lobes. Development of a pleural effusion — a collection of fluid between the surface of the diseased lung and the chest wall — is a not uncommon complication. Culture of the sputum will often serve to identify the bacterium and X-ray of the chest will confirm the presence and the site of the pneumonia and any pleural effusion present. The specific treatment of lobar (pneumococcal) pneumonia is Penicillin which is best given initially intramuscularly and later by mouth. Many such patients are gravely ill on admission to hospital and require expert nursing care with particular attention being paid to tepid sponging, relief of chest pain (best achieved by soluble aspirin) and provision of a liberal fluid intake and tolerable light diet. The response to penicillin is usually dramatic and the great majority of patients make a complete recovery, occasional fatalities occuring in the very young and the elderly.

Bronchopneumonia

As distinct from lobar pneumonia this disease process involves spread of infection commonly into both lungs, the damage not being confined by lobar boundaries. It is not due to only one infective agent but indeed may occur with a wide variety of organisms. In childhood, especially in infancy, the term bronchiolitis is used and in this age group the disease is frequently of viral origin. The other age group who tend to be attacked are the elderly and in them bacterial infection is often the cause of the illness. Again bacterial bronchopneumonia may supervene in any age group in the presence of a systemic viral infection such as influenza. Although in infants the onset is characteristically acute, older patients often experience the slower development of symptoms and hence in them the diagnosis may not be suspected for some time. A productive cough with purulent sputum is the main feature in the presentation of the illness. Physical signs may be minimal with only a few scattered crepitations audible over the lung fields or there may be widespread involvement with evidence of extensive consolidation. Occlusion of a bronchus with viscid secretions, leading to lung collapse, and the development of a lung abscess, are complications which must be recognised early in their development if appropriate management is to be effective in their correction. Examination of the sputum is an absolute necessity not only for precise diagnosis but as a guide to treatment since there is a wide variation in antibiotic sensitivity of the organisms commonly involved. X-ray examination of the chest is useful to determine more definitively the nature and extent of the disease, and presence of complications. Viral infections are unresponsive to antibiotics and hence must be treated symptomatically. Physiotherapy plays an important role in loosening and facilitating expectoration of bronchial secretions, and is particularly of importance in the treatment of complications, which only occasionally require surgical intervention. For bacterial infections appropriate antibiotics should be administered. Oxygen therapy may be required and supportive nursing care as for lobar pneumonia, constitutes a considerable part of management. Although many patients make an adequate recovery a notable proportion succumb from this illness, particularly those in the susceptible age groups who have pre-existing lung disease.

Pneumoconioses.

These are a group of chronic pulmonary diseases resulting from inhalation of mineral dusts, notably coal dust almost invariable in the course of the patients occupation, usually mining, and sharing the common feature of fibrosis of the lungs. Many years of environmental exposure to these dusts commonly elapse before the patient develops symptoms. Of these by far the most common is undue breathlessness on exertion which gradually becomes more severe until the patient is eventually breathless even at rest. Cough and wheezing may also occur. Some patients have little or no incapacity although their chest X-ray appearances are grossly abnormal. In certain of these diseases the affected patient is at an increased risk of developing pulmonary tuberculosis and even cancer of the lung, while others may suffer the complication of congestive cardiac failure. Physical features of note are the visible coexistence of dust particles in the skin, the presence of cyanosis and the over-inflated, barrel-shaped chest which has resulted from the development of emphysema. Clinical signs, such as ankle oedema, suggestive of other complications may be detectable. Since the lung damage is irreversible all attempts at prevention should be made. These ought to include the wearing of masks, the use of extractor fans and the wetting of atmospheric dust. Once the diagnosis has been made the patient should usually be advised to change his occupation. Some patients become reasonably accommodated to their disability while others deteriorate and die of respiratory failure or of a complication of the original disease.

Pulmonary Embolism.

Implied in the term is the obstruction to part or parts of the pulmonary blood flow by blood clots which have originated elsewhere in the circulation and which have been transported in the blood stream to the lungs, through which they cannot pass. The common sites from which such clots arise are the deep veins of the legs and the pelvic veins. These veins must themselves contain clots from which fragments break off to produce pulmonary embolism. If there is acute massive obstruction to the pulmonary circulation sudden death occurs. Short of this catastrophe there may result a spectrum of illness varying from the entirely asymptomatic to the moribund but potentially salvable. The commonest symptoms are sudden breathlessness and chest pain. A distinguishing feature of the former is that it may be alleviated by lying flat. Other symptoms such as haemoptysis are much less common. Low blood pressure and a rapid pulse rate are common findings and there may in addition be cyanosis and evidence of congestive cardiac failure. Clinical examination of the chest usually reveals no abnormality. Occasionally infarction of lung may occur — that is effective irreversible damage of that part of the lung beyond the site of obstruction. In this instance signs of pleurisy may be apparent. If the degree of circulatory obstruction is sufficient it may be apparent on a standard X-ray of chest. More precise diagnosis and localisation can be achieved by the technique of pulmonary angiography when X-rays of chest are taken after the injection of radio-opaque dye into the main pulmonary artery via a catheter introduced into an arm vein and passed through the right side of the heart. E.C.G. tracings may provide additional evidence to support the diagnosis. Treatment consists essentially of supportive measures such as elevation of the foot of the bed, if necessary, in an attempt to maintain the blood pressure and the administration of oxygen. Anti-coagulant therapy is usually advised hopefully with a view to reducing the likelihood of recurrence. Newer materials are available which may dissolve the clots but at present these remain to be fully assessed. If the patient survives the first few hours he is likely to complete his recovery. A few patients suffer recurrent episodes and as a result develop chronic lung disease which may precipitate congestive cardiac failure.

The Pleura

Pneumothorax

In this condition the surface of the lung and the inner chest wall which are normally in close contact, become separated by the presence of air between them. This situation may arise as a result of chest injury, or spontaneously, in association with an abnormality of the lung or its pleural surface. Varying degrees of lung collapse result, and may be complicated by the accumulation of blood or other fluids within the pleural cavity. Sudden chest pain and breathlessness constitute the main complaints. In most instances physical examination of the chest will reveal evidence of lung collapse and free air in the pleural space, findings which are readily confirmed on Chest X-ray. Most cases undergo spontaneous cure with absorption of the free air and re-expansion of the collapsed lung within two to three weeks. However if expansion does not occur spontaneously or if fluid collects within the pleural cavity drainage of the air and liquid should be effected through a catheter inserted into the pleural cavity. To minimise the risk of the introduction of infection by this manoeuvre the other end of the catheter is placed in a water seal. Occasional patients develop increasing tension of the air within the pleural space and they require emergency pleural drainage to avoid rapid deterioration in pulmonary function which may be fatal if the tension is unrelieved. A few patients suffer persistent lung collapse despite apparently adequate drainage. This then necessitates thoracotomy to bring about re-expansion.

Pleural Effusion

As a result of damage to the pleura it may produce an excessive amount of fluid which then accumulates within the pleural cavity and by compression of the underlying lung results in varying degrees of lung collapse. The pleural damage may be due to inflammation (pleurisy), involvement in tumour, or infarction of the underlying lung. Pleurisy commonly arises from lung infections such as lobar pneumonia or tuberculosis. Breathlessness and chest pain are the prominent symptoms, while there may be other complaints related to the underlying disease. Percussion over the affected region of the chest wall classically elicits extreme dullness and there may be additional signs of lung collapse. X-ray examination of the chest will in most instances serve to further define the nature of the problem, including any disease of the lung itself. Specific diagnosis can often be made by aspirating the pleural fluid through a needle, and examining it for evidence of the causal disease. This includes submitting specimens for bacteriological culture. Complete drainage of the pleural cavity should be performed if possible and the success of this procedure may be determined by subsequent Chest X-ray. Further treatment and prognosis depend almost entirely on correctly diagnosing the basic disease which has been responsible for producing the pleural damage. However if the fluid becomes heavily infected, resulting in the formation of an empyema, this will require individual appropriate antibiotic therapy and attention to drainage, and worsens the prognosis whatever the nature of the initial disease.

SPUTUM CHARACTERISTICS:

DISEASE	VOLUME	COLOUR	CONSISTENCY
Acute bronchitis	***	Yellow/green	Thick
Chronic bronchitis	**	White/grey	Thin
Bronchial asthma	*/−	White	Thick
Lobar pneumonia	**	Rust	Thin
Bronchiectasis	****	Yellow/green	Thick
Bronchopneumonia	***	Yellow/green	Thick
Pneumoconiosis	*	Grey/black	Thin
Pulmonary embolism	*/−	Red	Thick

3
Diseases of the Blood and Blood-Forming Organs

The Anaemias

Iron Deficiency Anaemia

The end result of the diminished availability of iron for blood formation, this situation usually results from blood loss but less commonly may be due to inadequate intake of iron in the diet or to one of the malabsorption syndromes. During pregnancy there is an increased requirement for iron. The severity of symptoms is usually related to the degree of anaemia, and the patient may be able to identify a source of blood loss such as menorrhagia or melaena. Weakness, tiredness, palpitations, headache and light headedness are common complaints. If the anaemia is sufficiently developed pallor of the mucous membranes is readily detectable. This is often most easily observed on the conjunctivae and tongue. Specific enquiry should be made about the precise composition of the diet and about possible routes of blood loss. Estimation of the haemoglobin concentration and the demonstration on a blood film of red cells with a low content of haemoglobin may strongly suggest the presence of iron deficiency which may be confirmed by measurement of the amount of iron in the blood.

Investigations will then need to be performed to search for a source of blood loss; in particular it is important to test for occult blood in the faeces and urine. A positive result will direct attention to the alimentary or urinary tracts which should then be subjected to appropriate further scrutiny to define the disease responsible for the blood loss, such as duodenal ulcer or tumours of the bowel or bladder. It is in most instances sufficient to administer iron salts in tablets by mouth. However if there is malabsorption or if the patient is intolerant of iron tablets, suffering for example abdominal pain after their administration, iron supplements may have to be given by intramuscular injection. Not infrequently, patients, usually women, fail to take the necessary tablets, and they too will require iron injections. If it is felt that they will be unlikely to complete a full course, then in selected cases it may be advisable to give the iron as a total intravenous dose. This procedure is not without some risk and is reserved for only a few patients. The anaemia of acute blood loss, especially when this is continuing or is associated with shock or some other complication will require correction by blood transfusion. Iron is necessary for a variety of other essential purposes within the body apart from its role in the formation of haemoglobin and it is consequently important to realise that although anaemia may be corrected quite quickly by administration of iron supplements these should be continued for some time thereafter to replenish the depleted body stores.

COMMON CAUSES OF IRON DEFICIENCY ANAEMIA	
1. Inadequate intake —	diet deficient particularly in animal meat
2. Malabsorption —	coeliac disease, post-gastric surgery
3. Blood loss —	menorrhagia, haematuria, haematemesis, malaise, epistaxis

Megaloblastic Anaemia

Encountered much less often than iron deficiency anaemia, this condition is almost always due to deficiency of either vitamin B_{12} or folic acid. The main natural source of vitamin B_{12} is meat and of folic acid is green vegetables. Dietary deficiency of vitamin B_{12} is rare since the body has large stores of this substance. Inadequate intake of folic acid however is not uncommon particularly when most of the vegetables consumed are previously cooked by boiling. Malabsorption is the main course of deficiencies of these vitamins. Combined deficiencies may occur in the various malabsorption syndromes while isolated malabsorption of vitamin B_{12} is encountered in pernicious anaemia, due to an abnormality in the stomach. In pregnancy the demands for folic acid are much increased and this may result in the development of a megaloblastic anaemia if the patient is not taking prophyllactic folic acid supplements. By the time the patient presents he is usually severely anaemic. In addition to the general symptoms of anaemia there is often the characteristic complaint of a painful tongue and if the anaemia is due to vitamin B_{12} deficiency there may be symptoms related to the spinal cord damage which classically accompanies some cases of this disease. These symptoms are very varied and include, weakness and tingling sensations in the limbs and loss of balance. Not only is the average patient markedly pale but in pernicious anaemia there may be a lemon yellow tint to the skin and mucous membranes. The tongue is frequently smooth and neurological examination may reveal objective evidence of spinal cord or peripherel nerve damage. The red blood cells are usually found to be larger than normal while estimation of the haemoglobin concentration will confirm the anaemia. Blood levels of vitamin B_{12} and folic acid may be measured and examination of the bone marrow will demonstrate that red cell formation is abnormal (in this case 'megaloblastic'). An augmented histamine test is performed if pernicious anaemia is suspected. In this condition the stomach fails to produce acid even after stimulation by histamine. Malabsorption of vitamin B_{12} can be established by the Schilling test in which radioactive vitamin B_{12} is given by mouth and a urine collection subsequently made to determine the proportion of vitamin which has been absorbed and excreted. Patients with pernicious anaemia absorb very little and hence only a very small amount is excreted in the urine.

Further tests of small bowel function, as described under the malabsorption syndrome, are required if there is a possibility of folic acid deficiency. Having established the precise diagnosis appropriate administration of vitamin B_{12} or folic acid should begin. Although folic acid is usually given by mouth, vitamin B_{12} must be given by injection for in pernicious anaemia if it is given orally insufficient quantities are absorbed. The response to treatment may be accurately assessed by serial measurements of the haemoglobin concentration and the reticulocyte count (the number of new red cells appearing in the circulation). The prognosis in pernicious anaemia is excellent while in folic acid deficiency due to malabsorption the outcome is largely determined by the nature of the disease affecting the small bowel.

It is vital that pernicious anaemia be distinguished from folic acid deficiency since administration of folic acid to patients with pernicious anaemia may result in the appearance or worsening of neurological damage which can be irreversible. Patients who have pernicious anaemia must of course continue to receive injections of vitamin B_{12} for the remainder of their lives.

Haemolytic Anaemia

For a variety of unrelated reasons red blood cells may undergo destruction (haemolysis) at an unduly rapid rate. If the bone marrow cannot respond sufficiently by producing enough new cells to compensate for the loss anaemia develops. Some conditions responsible for this phenomenon are inherited, while others are due to acquired diseases in many of which antibodies are developed by the patient against his own red cells. The common symptoms of anaemia are again encountered with the additional feature of jaundice in a proportion of patients. Physical examination serves to confirm these signs with the additional presence of an enlarged spleen often being disclosed. As would be anticipated an elevated reticulocyte count is characteristic of haemolytic anaemia and a variety of sophisticated investigations are available to pin-point the cause of the accelerated red cell destruction. Proper decisions on treatment require a precise diagnosis. In many instances there is no successful therapy while other situations lend themselves to treatment with steroid drugs or splenectomy.

Aplastic Anaemia

Complete or partial arrest of bone marrow function results in the formation of diminished numbers of blood cells. Approximately one half of patients affected have been exposed to a drug or other toxic agent which is recognised to produce this disastrous response. In the remainder no adequate explanation is available. Because of their low numbers of white blood cells such patients are highly susceptible to infections, while scarcity of platelets results in an undue tendency to bleed. These phenomena, combined with severe anaemia, account for the various ways in which patients with aplastic anaemia may present. On examination of the blood the pattern of diminished cell numbers can be appreciated while inspection of the bone marrow allows confirmation of its reduced function. Treatment consists largely of prevention and rapid attention to any infection and blood transfusion when symptoms of anaemia are sufficiently severe. A small number of patients appear to respond to large doses of male hormone but the remainder are fated to die of uncontrollable haemorrhage or overwhelming infection.

The Leukaemias

Acute Leukaemia

A malignant proliferation of white blood cells originating in the bone marrow and usually 'spilling over' into the blood, this disease may take one of several forms, denoted by the particular class of white blood cell involved. The cells which typify this situation are known as 'blasts'. Although considerable research has been performed in this field in recent years no definite agent has been shown to be the cause of this group of disorders. Symptoms tend to fall roughly into three groups — those related to infection, to anaemia and to undue bleeding. The malignant white cells have a reduced ability to combat infection, while characteristically affected patients are severely anaemic and suffer bleeding from mucosal surfaces and into the skin. Common clinical findings are pallor, bruising, enlarged lymph nodes and enlargement of the liver and spleen. Fever is a frequent sign and evidence of infection is often present. Careful examination of a blood film will usually serve to make the diagnosis which can be confirmed by study of the bone marrow, in which the profusion of abnormal cells may be identified. Children usually respond better to treatment than adults. Most patients are given steroids plus a variety of drugs which are intended to destroy the leukaemic cells. Blood transfusion is often required. Unfortunately although an initial success may be achieved in apparently clearing the leukaemic cells from the marrow, in virtually every instance a recurrence eventually occurs and a fatal outcome is almost inevitable.

Chronic Myeloid Leukaemia

Characterised by a massive increase in the total numbers of white blood cells, this form of leukaemia is much more common in adults than in children and most of the cells are mature in contradistinction to the primitive 'blasts' which typify the acute form of the disease. The great majority of patients have a highly specific chromosomal abnormality but no final cause has been established to account for the disorder. A notable number of patients are discovered to have the disease incidentally at routine blood examination, although the majority present with symptoms of anaemia or less often of infection. Physical findings are similar to those in acute leukaemia, although undue bleeding is less common and enlargement of the spleen is often very striking. Tenderness over the sternum is a characteristic feature. Again examination of the blood and bone marrow allows definition of the precise situation. The treatment of choice for chronic myeloid leukaemia is the drug Busulphan. Usually initial response is satisfactory and the anaemia resolves as the white blood count returns to normal levels. Despite this gratifying result eventual relapse occurs (often after a period of several years) and the features of acute leukaemia become evident heralding a rapid downhill course leading to death.

Chronic Lymphatic Leukaemia

Classically a disease of elderly patients this is a much more benign form of leukaemia than those previously discussed. Often the condition is discovered only accidentally or when the patient presents with enlargement of several groups of lymph nodes. A large liver and spleen are again typical findings. As with the other forms of leukaemia blood and bone marrow examination confirm the diagnosis. The course of the disease is often such that it does not shorten the life expectancy of those afflicted. Hence if the patient is without symptoms it is usually recommended that no treatment be given. When symptoms demand treatment the drug of first choice is generally accepted to be Chlorambucil which is almost always effective in bringing the white blood count to normal and in reducing the size of the various enlarged organs, often to their original dimensions, just as Busulphan does for patients with chronic myeloid leukaemia. Anaemia and undue bleeding however often only respond to the additional administration of steroids.

Other Malignant Diseases of the Blood Forming Organs

Polycythaemia Vera

In reality a process somewhat similar to chronic leukaemia, this disorder involves the red blood cells, in such a way that they become unduly numerous. As with the leukaemias no single cause has been demonstrated. Prominent symptoms are headache, undue breathlessness and generalised itch, which is especially troublesome after taking a bath.

In the characteristic patient there is a ruddy complexion, enlargement of the liver and spleen and mild hypertension. The haemoglobin concentration is high, often being more than 20 gms per 100 mls blood. A variety of techniques are available to confirm the presence of increased numbers of red blood cells. Initial treatment consists of removal by venesection of the quantity of blood in excess of normal. This is usually performed in stages over a period of about one week. Thereafter most patients receive a dose of radio-active phosphorous which is designed to reduce the rate of production of new red cells. With this form of management which usually has to be repeated at intervals, most patients will survive for 10 – 15 years, although some succumb earlier to complications such as cerebral or coronary thrombosis or the development of acute leukaemia.

Hodgkin's Disease

One of a group of disorders collectively known as the malignant lymphomas, this particular form tends to affect young adults. Once again the definite cause has not been established. The onset is usually slow with the appearance of an enlarged group of lymph nodes often in the region of the neck. These are classically painless and in the early stages may be the only evidence of the disease. If however the disease has progressed before the patient has sought medical advice more striking abnormalities may be found; several groups of nodes may be obviously involved, the liver and spleen are frequently enlarged and anaemia may have developed. The more advanced the disease, usually the more prominent the symptoms, with weakness, undue tiredness and observation of the enlarged organs being the main complaint. One characteristic but ill-understood symptom is that of pain in the limbs or trunk after taking alcohol. Diagnosis is usually firmly established by examination of biopsy material taken from one of the enlarged nodes.

If the patient presents at a stage when only one group of lymph nodes is involved, local radiotherapy is the treatment of choice. For the situations in which the disease is more widespread the administration of drugs aimed at destroying the malignant cells is usually advised. The earlier in the stage of his illness the patient presents, the better is the outlook. Occasional complete cures have occured, but more often the disease becomes progressively less responsive to treatment and spreads throughout the body with the anticipated fatal result.

Multiple Myeloma

This disease involves malignant proliferation of a type of cell known as the plasma cell, whose normal function seems to be the production of antibodies. The commonest presenting symptom is that of bone pain often accompanied by features of anaemia. Bony tenderness is a frequent finding and pathological fractures may even occur. Precise diagnosis is made by the identification of markedly increased number of plasma cells within the bone marrow, many of which are quite bizarre. Anaemia is usually confirmed and the E.S.R. is classically grossly elevated. X-ray examination will reveal the presence of bone destruction in many patients. Local radiotherapy is of considerable value in relieving bone pain while administration of the drug, Melphalan, by mouth is the method of choice for attempting to control the malignant process. Patients eventually die of infection or less often of renal failure within a period of a few months or years.

Bleeding Disorders

Purpura

A descriptive term applied to pinhead sized lesions on the skin and mucous membranes, representing tiny bruises, this disorder may result from diseases of the capillaries or from low numbers of blood platelets (thrombocytopenia) whose normal role is in the plugging of defects of which may occur in the small blood vessels. A variety of drugs have been blamed for producing each of these situations. However certain disease states may of themselves produce such abnormalities. An example of the former circumstance is scurvy in which, as a result of deficiency of Vitamin C, the capillaries are unduly fragile and rupture easily. Thrombocytopenia may occur in a wide variety of clinical situations varying in severity from measles to acute leukaemia. Purpura on the skin is rarely a problem but may be more serious when occuring in the eye or on mucous membranes such as in the alimentary tract. In these instances serious bleeding may occur. Methods of diagnosis will of course depend upon suspicion of the underlying problem and appropriate treatment will be determined by definition of the nature of that problem.

Haemophilia

With the related disorder, Christmas disease, this is the commonest hereditary defect in blood clotting. Because of the pattern of inheritance the illness is evident in the males while the females act as carriers for the abnormal gene which is responsible for the disease. Different individuals may suffer different degrees of severity of the clinical problems. The most severely affected boys have trouble from early childhood with bleeding into joints, extensive bruising, haematuria and much prolonged bleeding after dental extraction. The major difficulties experienced are a result of the recurrent joint haemorrhages. These produce severe pain and swelling with immobility of the affected joint and associated muscle wasting which contributes to further instability with consequent likelihood of further bleeds and eventual joint deformity. Treatment is directed to control of bleeding by infusing the patient with blood products which are rich in the clotting factor which he lacks. It is vital that such patients do not receive intramuscular injections nor oral aspirin, which may cause gastric bleeding even in patients who do not have a clotting defect. Skilled physiotherapy and orthopaedic management may play a considerable part in minimising joint damage and resultant complications. The disease is of course life long and affected individuals must learn to limit their activities to accommodate to their problem, and to attend hospital promptly should a bleeding episode occur.

4
Diseases of the Locomotor System

Rheumatoid Arthritis

An inflammatory process predominantly affecting the lining membrane of joints, the cause of this disease as yet eludes discovery despite the vast amount of research which has been performed. Although most of the clinical problem is related to joint involvement the disease is a generalised one and may affect many other organs and tissues. It usually begins in early adult life and is commoner in women than in men. Stiffness is the most common initial complaint and is often worst in the morning. Joint pain is characteristically worse when the affected joints are in use. These local symptoms are frequently accompanied by fatigue, weakness and weight loss particularly when many joints are involved. In the acute phase the joints are swollen, hot and tender and subcutaneous nodules may be found. Some patients suffer rapidly progressive damage with associated wasting of surrounding muscles and skin and subsequent severe crippling deformities, while others are more fortunate and only experience recurrent discomfort in a few joints with little functional disturbance. Many patients are moderately anaemic while an elevated E.S.R. is usually evidence of active disease.

Those patients who have a positive test for rheumatoid factor in the blood tend to have a worse prognosis. X-ray examination may reveal loss of joint space, osteoporosis of adjacent bone ends and punched out areas of bone erosion. Effective rest of the diseased joints is extremely important particularly in the acute phase when the application of local heat and graded physiotherapy are of considerable value. Aspirin is the drug of first choice and often effects considerable rapid relief of pain. Should this fail however, a variety of other agents are available in an effort to control symptoms. Steroid therapy should only be used as a last resort and then only after consultation with a physician who has a special interest in the management of this disease. Accurate splinting of acutely affected joints is an important manoeuvre to reduce the degree of subsequent deformity which in some individuals has necessitated surgical intervention. Recently surgical management of this disease has been advocated at an earlier stage in selected circumstances and appears to have met with some success.

Gout

This is a metabolic disorder which in its primary form is rarely seen in women but is not uncommon in men. The acute attack is due to the deposition of crystals of uric acid salts in the cartilage of joints. Classically the patient complains of a hot, swollen tender joint in his great toe. These features are readily confirmed on examination. The level of uric acid in the blood is commonly much elevated during such an episode. The great majority of cases undergo spontaneous cure or respond rapidly to appropriate treatment and do not recur. A few patients however suffer further attacks and develop chronic gout which may be complicated by renal damage. The acute attack is best treated by either Colchicine or Phenylbutazone. The former is a specific treatment for gout and is given as a 0·5mg tablet every two hours until cure is effected or the patient develops side effects, commonly diarrhoea. Chronic gout may be treated by a drug which prevents the build up of uric acid in the blood or by another which increases its excretion in the urine.

5
Diseases of the Pituitary

Anatomically and functionally this pea-sized organ which is sited at the base of the brain can be divided into two parts — anterior and posterior sections. In a general sense it serves to regulate to a large extent the function of the other hormone producing organs.

Acromegaly

Resulting from over production of growth hormone, this disease is usually due to a tumour arising from the anterior part of the gland. The fully developed clinical picture is quite characteristic with marked headache and often visual disturbance, enlargement of the head, hands and feet and thickening of the skin, being the main features. The diagnosis is essentially based on this clinical picture when it can be established that there has been a progression in the degree of organ enlargement. X-ray examination of the skull frequently reveals that the expanding tumour has eroded surrounding bone. If vision becomes impaired it is then necessary to remove surgically or destroy by irradiation the tumour itself and inevitably in addition the remainder of the gland. The onset of the disease is usually in middle age and affected patients commonly have a normal life expectancy.

Hypo-pituitarism

While arising from a wide spectrum of underlying causes varying from fractures of the base of the skull to tumours of the gland or surrounding structures, the end result in this disorder is partial or complete failure of function predominantly of the anterior part of the gland. In adults the commonest cause is infarction of the gland following post-partum haemorrhage. The onset of symptoms thereafter is usually slow with failure of lactation, lack of further menstruation, personality changes and features of thyroid and adrenal insufficiency. Physical findings include pale, smooth, fine skin with loss of pubic and axillary hair and low blood pressure. A battery of highly sophisticated investigations are available to help confirm the diagnosis and unravel the magnitude of the effect of the pituitary insufficiency on the other dependant endocrine glands. As is only too evident replacement of the missing hormones or use of suitable substitutes is essential. It is most important to provide Cortisone and Thyroxine to restore as far as possible the role of the adrenal and thyroid glands. The greatest danger to life is from acute adrenal failure. Once regular maintenance supplements have been established however a good prognosis is more or less assured.

Diabetes Insipidus

One of the main functions of the posterior part of the pituitary is to produce a hormone which plays an important part in regulating water balance. This hormone acts on the kidney to induce it to conserve water. When for any reason this part of the gland is damaged or destroyed the kidney is no longer under the influence of this antidiuretic hormone, fails to retain adequate fluid and so continuous high output of urine occurs. It is this complaint which brings the patient to seek advice, for he may pass up to 20 litres of urine in 24 hours, with of course a similar volume of fluid intake. By a variety of manoeuvres it can be shown whether the posterior part of the gland is working normally in this respect. If it is demonstrated to be deficient replacement therapy with intramuscular injections of Pitressin should be instituted. The great danger to these patients is naturally that of dehydration but with control of urine volume with appropriate amounts of Pitressin the risk is greatly reduced.

6
Diseases of the Thyroid

Acting mainly to control the rate of the great number of metabolic processes within various organs this gland when diseased may produce too little or too much hormones resulting in the appearance of usually readily identifiable clinical illnesses.

Hyperthyroidism (Thyrotoxicosis)

When the gland, for as yet incompletely understood reasons, manufactures excess thyroid hormones the various phases of metabolism under its influence become accelerated. Common complaints are then of increased sweating, irritability and nervousness, palpitations, increased appetite, loss of weight, intolerance of heat and often undue prominence of the eyes (exophthalmos). Examination

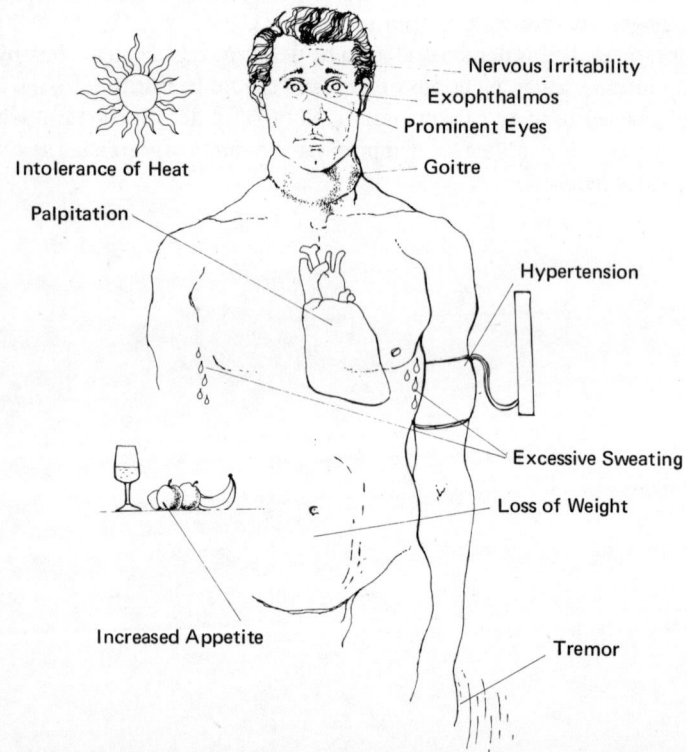

usually reveals a patient unable to relax, talkative, anxious and tremulous. The heart rhythm may be that of atrial fibrillation and there is frequently mild hypertension. Objective confirmation of the other symptoms is readily made. In the majority of patients the thyroid gland is visibily and palpably enlarged and indeed this may be the feature which has induced patients to seek medical advice. Rarely the exaggerated metabolic activity may bring the patient to the brink of exhaustion and at risk of death. Since thyroid hormones contain iodine, estimation of the amount of iodine in the blood and of the amount used by the hyperactive thyroid gland will allow demonstration of the increased amount and rate of production of the hormones. Broadly speaking there are three possible lines of treatment to attempt to control the amount of hormones produced by the gland, and there are fairly well defined indications for each. A variety of drugs whose function is to reduce the availability of iodine for hormone production, often prove effective. In some situations surgical removal of most of the gland is advised, while in older patients the gland may be to a large extent destroyed by radioactive iodine. Unfortunately all of these methods have risks and failures and these to a large extent determine the eventual outcome of the disease.

Hypothyroidism.

While diminished thyroid hormone production may be the result of unexplained gland failure or its involvement in an inflammatory process, it is nowadays encountered all too commonly following treatment of hyperthyroidism especially by sub-total thyroidectomy or radioactive iodine. As might be anticipated the clinical features are to a large extent the reverse of those of hyperthyroidism. In the great majority of instances the disease is of insidious onset and may go unrecognised for years. There is general slowing of physical and mental activity with the development of voice hoarseness, thickening and coarsening of the skin, tongue and hair and increase in body weight with diminished appetite and constipation, while a slow heart rate and effort angina are common additional manifestations. Like most diseases of the thyroid gland this disorder is commoner in women and a notable number of those affected undergo a premature menopause. Again, measurement of blood iodine and the utilization of iodine by the thyroid serve as accurate estimates of the diminished thyroid function. To restore normality replacement therapy with thyroid hormone is required. This should always be started at a low dose such as 0.05 mgs. Thyroxine per day and only slowly increased at intervals of approximately two weeks, particularly in those patients who have angina, to avoid precipitating cardiac failure or myocardial infarction. The eventual maintenance dose of Thyroxine is usually of the order of 0.2 mgs. per day which of course must be continued for life. The actual maintenance dose is determined entirely by the clinical response.

7
Diseases of the Adrenals

Like the pituitary the adrenal glands may each be considered anatomically and functionally in two parts. Each is situated close to the upper pole of the kidney on the same side. The outer shell of each gland constitutes its cortex and produces a variety of hormones which play important roles in the metabolism of salt and water and carbohydrate, and in the development of secondary sexual characteristics. The core of each gland is the medulla which manufactures substances which act on the several parts of the nervous system facilitating the transmission of nerve impulses.

Cushing's Syndrome.

Over production of hormones from the adrenal cortex may be due to a number of different factors. There may be a tumour in the pituitary gland which produces adrenocorticotrophic hormone (A.C.T.H.) whose action is to stimulate the cells of the adrenal cortex. This is the commonest cause of Cushing's syndrome in adults. Alternatively the primary abnormality may lie in the adrenal glands themselves in the form of a benign or malignant tumour. A situation very similar to Cushing's syndrome and met with much more commonly is that induced by the administration of steriod drugs such as Prednisone in a high dose for a prolonged period of time. Whatever the basic cause the result is a patient who presents with weakness, obesity, a round face, depression and often backache. Characteristically such patients have a moon-shaped face which is florid and often affected by acne. The trunk is usually markedly obese often in contrast to the limbs and classically there are purple striae on the hips and abdominal wall. Hypertension is a frequent accompanying feature. By measurement of the hormones and their breakdown products in the blood and urine it is possible to confirm the clinical diagnosis while further complex biochemical investigations will help to decide the nature of the underlying disorder. Once the diagnosis has been established with certainty it is then in order to proceed to surgically remove the tumour in the adrenal gland or more commonly most of both adrenals when there is a pituitary tumour. Thereafter steroid supplements are usually required for life. If the patient can be carefully brought to this stage in management he can usually look forward to a normal life expectancy.

Addison's Disease.

The reverse of Cushing's syndrome this disorder reflects failure of the adrenal cortex to produce adequate amounts of its hormones. The glands may for some poorly understood reason simply fail to function or they may be involved in other diseases such as secondary carcinoma or tuberculosis. Again the adrenal glands may have been removed not just for Cushing's syndrome but for instance in an attempt to control cancer of the breast. Unfortunately adrenal failure may not uncommonly result from too sudden withdrawal of steroid therapy particularly when high doses of the drug have been used over prolonged periods. The full blown clinical situation is of a weak, wasted patient with an unduly pigmented skin and low blood pressure who has recurrent episodes of nausea, vomiting and diarrhoea. Personality disorders may be outstanding. The lack of control of salt and water balance constitutes a grave risk and may in many patients leads to an emergency situation which is commonly fatal if not recognised. Measurement of the blood electrolytes serves to confirm the imbalance and again analysis of blood and urine for the various hormones will afford an accurate means of determination of the state of adrenal function. Perhaps the best test in this context is that in which the adrenals are stimulated by an injection of A.C.T.H. The degree of their response in terms of hormone production provides a good assessment of their functional ability. The emergency situation of adrenal crisis referred to must be treated by infusion of saline and administration of hydrocortisone. In addition since most of these patients have low blood sugars supplements of dextrose are required. Thereafter maintenance therapy for life is necessary. Usually two drugs are required, one largely to restore normal carbohydrate metabolism and the other to maintain water and electrolyte balance. Attention must of course be paid to any remediable underlying disease such as tuberculosis. Once normal metabolic balance has been achieved the prognosis is good but may be altered by the nature of the basic cause, for example secondary carcinoma.

Phaeochromocytoma.

A tumour arising usually from the adrenal medulla, this is one of the rarer causes of hypertension. Prominent symptoms are headache, palpitations, sweating and diarrhoea. The hypertension is often, at least in the early stages, intermittent and the symptom complex tends to occur with elevations of the blood pressure. Most of the clinical features can be attributed to the excessive amount of adrenaline and noradrenaline, the hormones secreted by the tumour, for they induce changes in the heart and blood vessels which result in the production of high blood pressure. Levels of these hormones and their metabolites may be measured in the blood and urine and in this disease they are found to be greatly increased. The tumour may be localised by highly sophisticated X-ray examinations and thereafter must be removed surgically. Control of the blood pressure before, during and after operation requires considerable skill and close observation. Providing that the patient has presented before hypertension has become established and largely irreversible and if he can be brought through the difficult phase surrounding operation the outlook is favourable.

8
Diseases of the Pancreas

Diabetes Mellitus

Although the story of diabetes mellitus involves much more than the pancreas it is convenient to consider the disease at this juncture since the pancreas is the site of production of the hormone insulin which is deficient or relatively ineffective in diabetes. Similarly there are many more aspects to the disease than high levels of blood sugar (hyperglycaemia), although this remains the diagnostic hallmark of the condition. In some diabetics it appears that there is a true deficiency of insulin, that is the pancreas fails to produce sufficient quantities for the metabolic needs of the body, but in a large number of patients the amount of insulin produced is quite normal or even in excess of normal and yet its action seems to be impeded. The features of diabetes mellitus in one form or another affect a suprisingly large proportion of the adult population, possibly as much as 5%.

The classical presenting complaints especially in young adults are of polyuria, polydipsia (increased thirst) and loss of weight. There may in addition be a multitude of other symptoms such as itching, pins and needles and diarrhoea. One of the commonest forms however is in the middle aged or elderly patient with obesity and hypertension who is found on routine examination to have sugar in the urine (glycosuria). Unfortunately diabetes is virtually characterised by its complications which seem to arise either from the hyperglycaemia e.g. (susceptibility to infections) or from the thickening and narrowing of the small blood vessels throughout the body which is a common feature of this disease and may be visualised at ophthalmoscopic examination. In various ways there may follow damage to the eye and brain, to the heart and peripheral arteries (particularly in the leg), to the spinal cord and peripheral nerves and to the kidneys. Hence infections in the skin, chest and urinary tract, several forms of blindness cerebrovascular accidents, claudication and gangrene, hypertension, myocardial infarction and heart failure; peripheral neuropathy, and renal insufficiency and nephrotic syndrome are met with all too frequently in

Complications of Diabetes

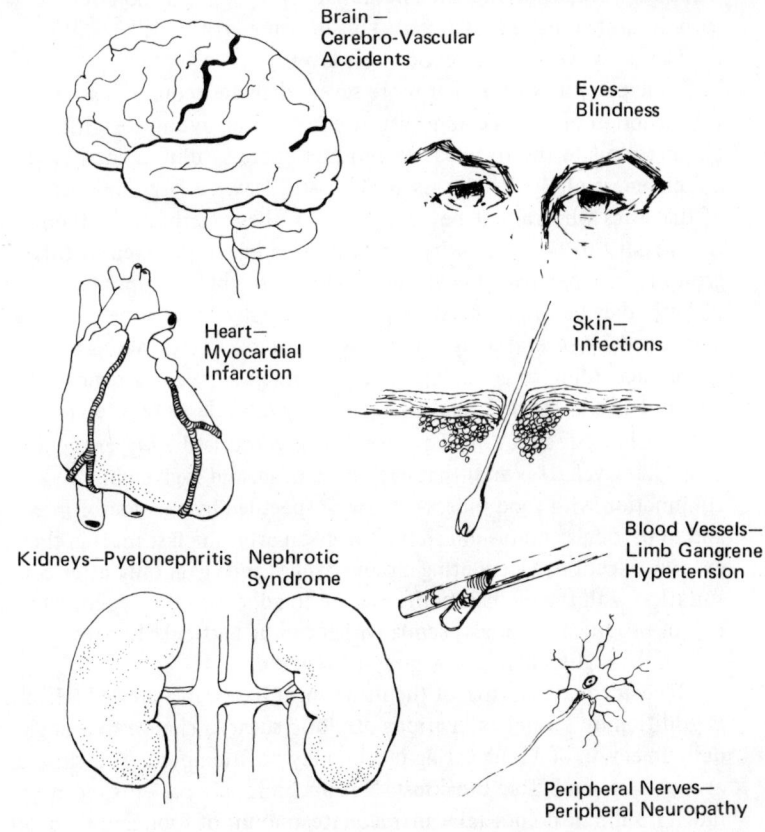

the diabetic patient and of themselves may pose diagnostic and therapeutic difficulties. The simplest and surest way to firmly establish the diagnosis is by the oral glucose tolerance test, during which the fasting blood sugar level should be greater than 120 mgs.% and the level at some other stage in the test (which lasts 2½ hours) greater than 180 mgs.%. Depending on the severity of the disorder the regime of management will fall into one of three main categories. Firstly dietary control alone; usually applicable to the obese older patient with mild diabetes. Total calorie intake and in particular consumption of carbohydrate must be restricted. This measure is often sufficient to control body weight and blood sugar levels.

Some patients with rather more severe diabetes require in addition to restriction of diet the administration of a drug by mouth which will either stimulate the pancreas to produce more insulin or increase the effectiveness of the insulin itself. This still leaves a large number of diabetics who cannot be controlled by these methods. In them it is necessary to use insulin by subcutaneous injection. Even in this group it is imperative that strict adherence to the appropriate diabetic diet be imposed. Such patients initially have to be controlled by several daily injections of soluble (quick acting) insulin according to a 'sliding scale' by which is meant a regime of doses of insulin graded to the degree of glycosuria as registered in the 'Clinitest' situation. The more the glycosuria the bigger the dose of insulin given. It is vital that each dose of insulin is given in conjunction with food unless otherwise specified by the doctor in charge and in particular no insulin should be given after the last meal in the evening except in extenuating circumstances and again only after consultation with the medical staff. Failure to adhere to this regime runs the risk of producing hypoglycaemia which can be particularly dangerous during the night when it may go unrecognised.

Once adequate control of the urine sugar has been achieved (checked in addition by several estimations of blood sugar) a change to a single daily injection of a long acting insulin may be attempted. This should always be given before breakfast. Not uncommonly patients receive too much insulin or do not take an adequate amount of food and then develop hypoglycaemia. Early symptoms are a feeling of hunger and apprehension, followed by sweating and eventual alteration of consciousness which may progress through abnormal behaviour to frank coma. Should a patient develop such symptoms he must be given a glucose drink, if he is conscious, or an intravenous injection of glucose if he is unconscious. The rapid recovery which subsequently occurs confirms the diagnosis. Less often the balance becomes upset in the opposite direction and the blood sugar rises to very high levels accompanied by other highly dangerous biochemical abnormalities. This situation usually arises from the patients failure to take adequate amounts of insulin or from the development of a superimposed infection. The onset is gradual with progressive drowsiness, overbreathing, exhalation of acetone in the breath and finally coma. Management is complicated and time consuming and must be matched by close serial observation of the patient's pulse, blood pressure, respiratory rate, fluid balance and level of consciousness apart from the numerous biochemical investigations.

Co-operation between the medical and nursing staff is of great importance for a notable number of patients who have suffered this emergency situation have died at least in part as a result of bad management. When the time comes for the diabetic to leave hospital he must be intimately instructed in the care and use of his syringe and insulin and the technique of urine testing. It must be emphasised that dietary control plays a major part in the treatment of his disease and he should be advised to report any change in his condition immediately. On leaving hospital his requirements for insulin will be less than the dose he was receiving during his admission for he will be returning to a life of greater activity and effectively 'burning up' more carbohydrate. Apart from the hazards of hyperglycaemic and hypoglycaemic coma, strict control of the blood sugar levels unfortunately does not protect the diabetic from developing the complications of his disease and it is usually of one of these complications that he finally succumbs though most patients can look forward to many years of fruitful existance before this eventuality.

9
Diseases of the Kidneys

Acute Pyelonephritis.

An inflammatory disease of the kidneys frequently associated with infection by organisms commonly found in the colon, there is a variety of circumstances which predispose to its development. These include obstruction and instrumentation of the urinary tract, infancy, pregnancy and neurological disorders of the bladder. Women are affected much more commonly than men and at least in part this appears to be due to the relative closeness of the female anal and urethral orifices, so that organisms from the bowel may more readily enter the lower urinary tract. The common presentation is with sudden onset of symptoms of fever accompanied by pain in the loins, burning discomfort on passing urine and an increased frequency of micturition. Usually there is tenderness in the loins and often over the bladder area. The urine can be shown to contain pus cells and organisms. The precise nature of these is determined by culture of a mid-stream specimen. This procedure will also reveal the range of antibiotics or sulphonamide drugs to which the particular organism is sensitive. Treatment consists specifically of administration of the appropriate drug to eradicate the infection. A highly important supportive measure is the provision of a liberal fluid intake, in excess of three litres per day in an adult patient, if this can be tolerated. Such a regime is essential when the patient is receiving a sulphonamide since this group of drugs have a tendency to cause urinary obstruction and even acute renal failure. In addition the high urinary output which will result from an increased fluid intake has a flushing effect on the kidneys. The great majority of attacks respond rapidly to this form of management.

Acute Glomerulonephritis.

As a result of an allergic response to a specific organism — the streptococcus — a small number of patients, usually young children, develop an inflammatory disease of those parts of the kidneys which are responsible for filtering the blood. This reaction commonly develops ten to fourteen days after a throat infection, the patient then complaining of swelling of the feet and ankles, puffiness of the face,

Signs of Glomerulonephritis

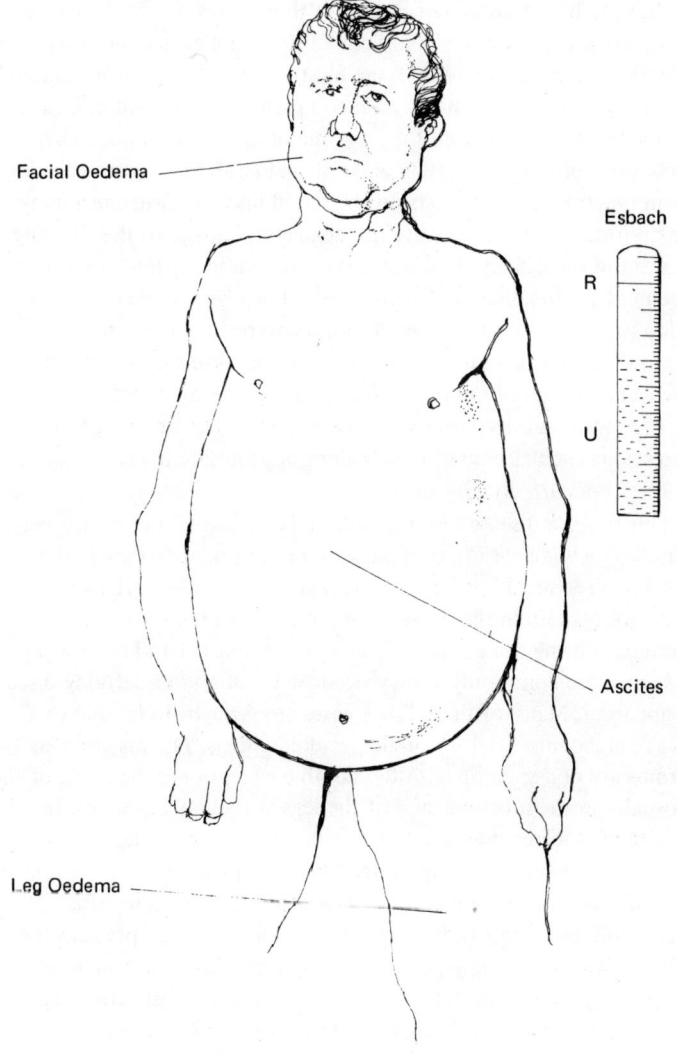

headache, reduced urine volume and the passage of blood in the urine. Physical examination will confirm the presence of oedema and further reveal that the blood pressure is raised. If there is severe renal damage, visual disturbances, cardiac failure, convulsions and even coma may occur. Some patients during the initial stage fail to respond to treatment, rapidly deteriorate and die. A few make an incomplete recovery and continue to suffer renal damage, although the great majority return to normality. The urine contains blood and protein and a throat swab may demonstrate the organism on culture, while tests on the blood may confirm the allergy to the streptococcus and indicate the degree of damage to the filtering mechanism in the kidney. Bed rest constitutes an important part in the management of this illness. Penicillin should be given to clear any throat infection present and it is usually necessary to restrict the intake of fluids, protein, salt and potassium until the kidney function spontaneously improves. The raised blood pressure may on occasion be sufficiently severe to require anti-hypertensive therapy, while the treatment of complications such as convulsions is along appropriate lines.

The Nephrotic Syndrome.

This is not a disease but a collection of abnormalities which may be caused by a wide variety of diseases. The abnormalities are — the presence of oedema, a low level of protein in the blood, and a very high level of protein in the urine. This group of findings may be encountered during the course of some rather unusual and interesting diseases or more commonly it may occur without any underlying disease being apparent. Many of these latter cases are thought to be due to a previous unrecognised attack of glomerulonephritis. The majority of symptoms are non-specific with the notable exception of swelling of the face, usually in the morning, and of the legs as the day advances. In some patients the accumulation of excess fluid in the tissues may be severe. The presence of oedema is readily confirmed on examination. Biochemical analysis of the blood will confirm the characteristic findings while the various tests available to determine the presence of proteinuria will be strongly positive. A fairly accurate test to measure the amount of protein in the urine involves the use of Esbach's reagent. In the classical case this will register a result of $5 - 20$ parts that is $5 - 20$ gms. per litre of urine. To obtain a precise diagnosis of the nature of the underlying disease, a renal biopsy will be necessary. Apart from losing protein in the urine, most of the patients, at least initially, have otherwise normal renal function, but they are unduly susceptible to infections. As long as renal function remains satisfactory a high protein diet should be given i.e. 120 – 150 gms. protein per day. Salt intake should be restricted to a bare minimum. Some patients, mostly children, respond dramatically to steriod therapy while a few may become worse. If the oedema does not resolve with steriods diuretic therapy is indicated. Patients who do not recover slowly enter a phase of chronic renal failure.

Acute Renal Failure.

A complication which may arise in a wide variety of diseases, this emergency situation is usually accompanied by a markedly diminished urinary output (less than 500 mls. per day). Initially there may be no symptoms and the diagnosis is only suspected by measurement of the urine volume. Later, as a result of the retention in the blood of waste products and other materials, consequent on the poor renal function, a number of non specific symptoms may occur, including loss of appetite and well-being, weakness and undue sleepiness, One of the most important additional features readily appreciated on examination is that of fluid retention especially in the lungs and dependent parts. Highly significant abnormalities are detectable in the urine, such as low specific gravity with excess protein and blood, while analysis of the blood allows an accurate assessment of the damaging results of renal failure in terms of the presence and amounts of the numerous substances whose excretion is impaired. Conservative management is usually indicated in the first instance. Frequent regular recording of such information as urine volume, blood pressure and body weight is essential. Protein, salt and potassium (in the form of fruit and fruit juices) are excluded from the diet and fluid intake is severely restricted.

More specific measures may have to be taken to combat dangerous results of renal failure such as high blood potassium levels and excessive fluid retention. If despite this regime there is no improvement resort to peritoneal or haemodialysis may have to be made. The latter procedure in particular requires a high degree of skill and experience and can only be performed in a specialised unit. Superimposed infection and a tendency to undue bleeding constitute common hazards in the course of this illness. The eventual outcome in any individual is determined by the nature of the underlying disease, the promptness of diagnosis and the speed and skill with which the appropriate management is put into effect.

Chronic Renal Failure.

The end result of persistent, long standing kidney damage, this ailment is imposing an ever increasing load on the resources of the health services as facilities for long term haemodialysis and renal transplantation become more widely available, in response to public demand and necessity. Chronic glomerulonephritis and chronic pyelonephritis probably account for the great majority of cases of chronic renal failure. Common presenting symptoms are lassitude and apathy with generalised weakness. Headache, loss of appetite, nausea, vomiting, diarrhoea and itching in the skin constitute frequent complaints. Many patients have pale mucous membranes and hyperpigmented skin. Hypertension and oedema are often encountered and in the advanced stages a bleeding tendency, muscle twitching and even frank convulsions may be seen. The degree of impairment of renal function may be assessed by measurement of the urine specific gravity and daily urine volume and by estimation of accumulated waste products in the blood such as urea and creatinine. Most patients with chronic renal failure are notably anaemic probably in large part as a result of depression of the bone marrow by the accumulated waste products, and this additional feature makes a significant contribution to their illness. A high proportion of these patients require to restrict their dietary protein intake and as the degree of renal failure increases, their intake of salt and water as well. Severely affected individuals, if suitable candidates, may be kept alive by regular haemodialysis, usually performed twice per week, but this procedure in no sense offers a cure, for the problem can only finally be solved by successful renal transplantation.

10
Diseases of the Heart and Blood Vessels

Rheumatic Fever and Valvular Heart Disease.

Organic disease of the heart valves is most frequently the result of damage sustained during an episode of acute rheumatism (rheumatic fever). Approximately 25% of patients who suffer an attack of rheumatic fever will eventually, after an interval of often more than ten years, develop permanent abnormalities in the heart valves. Rheumatic fever commonly develops one to two weeks after a streptococcal sore throat and seems to be a consequence of allergy to the infecting organism. The connective tissues of the body become involved in an inflammatory process which particularly affects the joints, heart, skin and brain. Most patients are in the age group 5 – 15 years, while the disease is especially common in circumstances of cold, damp and overcrowding. Joint pains are a striking feature. The pain appears to move from joint to joint, often flaring up and subsiding in a few days in each joint involved.

Fever is a common accompanying feature and less often there may in addition be a skin rash, nodules under the skin and chorea, a disturbing involuntary movement disorder. The joints may be hot, swollen and tender and mobility is often greatly restricted. A rapid pulse is an almost constant feature, the heart may be palpably enlarged and there may be various murmurs suggesting that the valves, the heart muscle or its outer covering, the pericardium, are inflamed. The white blood cell count and E.S.R. are characteristically elevated and an E.C.G. and Chest X-ray will confirm the nature and degree of the heart involvement. Of considerable value in clinching the diagnosis is the A.S.O. titre which is an index of the body's response to streptococcal infections. Because of the hypersensitivity thought to exist in this area in rheumatic fever the values obtained are often very high. A throat swab will often allow identification of the causal organism. The principles of treatment comprise eradication of infection, suppression of the inflammation and resting the damaged tissues. To these ends Penicillin is prescribed, initially by the intramuscular route and later orally to kill the streptococcus. Aspirin is used with the aim of reducing the inflammatory process; and complete bed rest is enforced in the early stages of the illness. It is important to administer sufficiently large doses of aspirin even of the order of 10 gms. or more per day. Apart from the observable clinical response the best indicator of rheumatic activity is the E.S.R. which falls progressively with improvement. The great majority of patients make a complete recovery in the first instance. To prevent recurrences it is advisable for the patient to continue low dose oral Penicillin daily till he is well out of the vulnerable teenage period.

Features of Rheumatic Fever

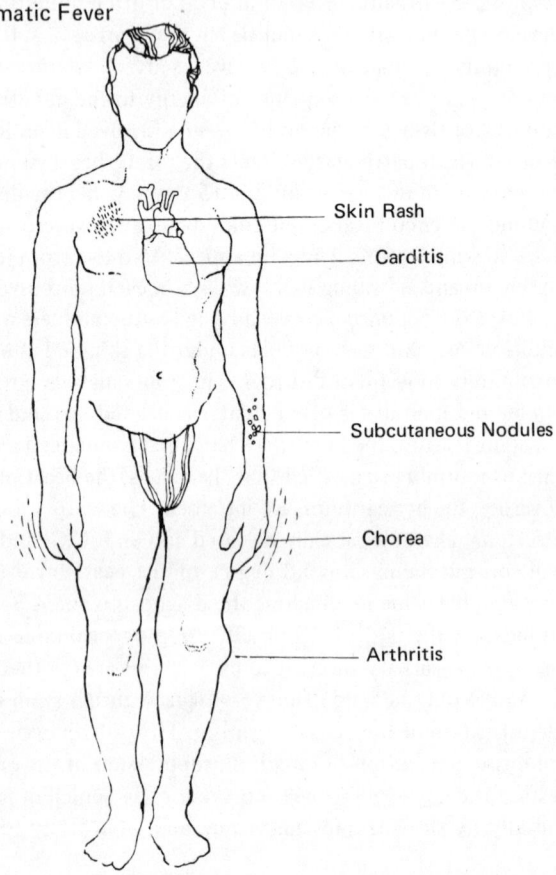

When irreversible damage to the heart valves occurs it becomes manifest as stenosis or incompetence or both. A stenosed valve is one which fails to open completely and so forms an obstruction to the passage of blood through its aperture. An incompetent valve on the other hand fails to close completely and therefore allows leakage of blood to occur in a direction opposite to that of normal flow. The valve most commonly affected by these forms of damage is the mitral valve which separates the left ventricle from the left atrium. Because of the increased load which these defects impose, the heart has to work harder to achieve the same effect as a normal heart. Hence early symptoms of valvular heart disease are palpitations and undue tiredness. The progressively increasing load however often proves too much for the heart which begins to fail with the resulting development of breathlessness and ankle swelling. Haemoptysis is a common complaint particularly in mitral stenosis and is usually due to pulmonary congestion. Severely disabled patients may be cyanosed, while further physical examination often reveals evidence that heart failure is present such as distended neck veins and an enlarged tender liver. Detailed examination of the heart first by palpation and subsequently by auscultation often allows a fairly precise diagnosis to be made in terms of which valves are involved, the nature of the damage and the effect of the damage on the separate chambers of the heart. Again a plain chest X-ray and E.C.G. are helpful confirmatory investigations. In some patients in whom doubt remains concerning the nature of the valve damage, more sophisticated procedures such as cardiac catheterisation have to be invoked to unravel the complexities of diagnosis. Most patients, at least in the early phase of the disease are managed conservatively with advice on restriction of effort and treatment of cardiac failure as required.

A minority of patients are suitable candidates for cardiac surgery. Unfortunately in many instances the individual's disability tends to be progressive with treatment becoming less and less effective. Complications occur all too frequently. The most important of these are subacute bacterial endocarditis and cerebral embolism. The former is basically an infection of the already damaged heart valves due to the presence of an organism within the cirulation. Further damage results and heart function deteriorates. Many patients succumb from this situation which requires aggressive treatment in the form of high dose long term antibiotics and support for the failing heart. Cerebral embolism is often encountered as a complication of valvular heart disease. The thrombus from which the embolus arises is usually sited in the left atrium where it has accumulated as a result of stagnation of blood in this chamber due most commonly to mitral stenosis. Hemiplegia is the characteristic outcome and skilled persistent physiotherapy is required to overcome the locomotor deficit. It is generally recommended that a patient who has suffered this set-back should receive anti-coagulant drugs in an effort to prevent the further deposition of thrombus and the risk of recurrent embolism.

Coronary artery disease.

Confined largely to populations in the developed countries, the essential feature of this condition is irregular narrowing of the arteries which supply the heart muscle. Although no causal factors have been definitely established to account for the abnormalities which appear in these blood vessels, it seems that cigarette smoking and the composition of the diet play major roles in the development of the disease. As a result of diminution in the calibre of the vessels involved the blood supply to the heart is impaired (myocardial ischaemia). If the disease becomes sufficiently advanced the blood supply to an area of heart muscle may be completely shut off. This results in death of that part, a process known as myocardial infarction. The final complete occlusion of a coronary artery may be due to thrombosis. Patients who suffer from this disease may initially have no symptoms. When symptoms develop they are usually in the nature of angina of effort. On exercise the patient experiences a dull pain commonly in the centre of the chest which may radiate to the neck or the arms. Lack of oxygen for normal heart muscle function is the basic cause of the pain and is of course a reflection of the reduced blood supply, which becomes more evident when the increased demands of exercise are imposed on the heart.

As the disease advances the patient can tolerate less and less exercise. The heart may eventually become so chronically short of oxygen that it begins to fail. A more dramatic event is the occurence of a myocardial infarction. In this situation chest pain is usually severe and unlike the pain of angina is characteristically not relieved by rest. The onset is classically sudden and frequently accompanied by profuse sweating, vomiting and even loss of consciousness. Frank heart failure may occur. While there are virtually no physical signs detectable in most patients with myocardial ischaemia, the reverse is often the case when infarction supervenes. Many patients are clinically shocked with pale cold even cyanosed extremities, a rapid feeble pulse, sweating, low blood pressure and impairment of consciousness. The E.C.G. is the most useful technique for determining the extent of myocardial ischaemia and the presence and site of actual infarction. Estimations in the blood of heart muscle enzymes which have leaked from the damaged tissue give additional useful information. A notable proportion of such patients have a transient fever which is thought to represent an aspect of the body's response to death of part of the heart muscle. The management of angina of effort is directed towards limitation of pain and hopeful prevention of infarction. Patients who are obese are advised to lose weight, work and exercise should be restricted below the limits which are known in the individual to provoke pain and cigarette smoking is discouraged. A variety of drugs from Glyceryl trinitrate to Propranolol are available for use in attempts to reduce angina. They may act in several different ways but do not to any appreciable extent dilate the narrowed coronary arteries.

Myocardial infarction frequently poses an emergency problem, which demands considerable skill in its management for complications are common and often difficult to control. In the section on specific nursing management of myocardial infarction are detailed the several important points related to the care of these patients. Failure to adhere to these principles can have severe adverse consequences. Relief of pain is essential. Powerful analgesics such as Heroin are employed and may require to be administered on several occasions. Inhalational oxygen therapy is of considerable benefit to many patients. Frequent monitoring of the various vital parameters is crucial to good management for alterations in therapy may be determined by changes in these measurements. Certain selected patients may be candidates for anticoagulant therapy, close supervision of which is a critical part of the nurse's duty. Heart failure will require additional appropriate management while the complications of cardiogenic shock and cardiac arrest often require highly specialised therapeutic techniques. The prompt recognition by the nurse of the latter situation and her rapid response is in most instances the most important factor instrumental in the patient's recovery. The characteristic features are usually obvious with loss of consciousness, absence of palpable pulse and audible heart sounds, and progressive dilation of the pupils. Immediate attention of other members of staff should be drawn as quickly as possible, a patent airway established and artificial ventilation synchronised with external cardiac massage begun. The chances of the patient's survival as already indicated are closely related to the rapidity and efficiency with which these manoeuvres are put into effect. There is a significant mortality rate from myocardial infarction, of the order of 20 – 25%. Most of the deaths occur in the first few hours following the event. A certain number of surviving patients may be incapacitated by heart failure, angina of effort or one of a number of other complications. Nevertheless a notable proportion made an uneventful recovery and if they adhere to the advice offered on sensible restriction of activity, may return to a useful existence.

Hypertension.

The normal level of blood pressure for healthy individuals rises with increasing age. Hypertension is the existence of a blood pressure above the acceptable upper limit of normal for age. For most adults this upper limit of normal is arbitrarily taken to be 140/90 mms. Hg. Of all patients seen with the common feature of an elevated blood pressure, only in some 15% can an underlying cause be found. These constitute the examples of secondary hypertension while the remaining majority are said to have primary or essential hypertension. Most of the secondary cases are due to kidney disease while a few are a result of much less common disorders arising in other organs such as the adrenals and thyroid gland (see Cushing's syndrome, phaeochromocytoma and thyrotoxicosis). Many patients with hypertension have rather vague symptoms such as lethargy, tiredness and diminished ability to concentrate. Headache may be prominent, and palpitations, undue breathlessness, light headedness and reduced visual acuity are frequent complaints. Nocturia may be a troublesome feature. These manifestations all reflect effects on the heart, brain and kidney from the changes in the small blood vessels associated with the high pressure within them. Should these effects become severe the clinical phenomena of angina of effort, myocardial infarction, strokes, heart or kidney failure may become apparent. Numerous hypertensive patients are overweight and many are psychoneurotic. Physical examination should be directed towards assessing the effects of the high blood pressure on the various vulnerable organs. Hence there may be evidence of heart enlargement or even failure, of previous strokes or of disease in the optic fundi, where the small blood vessels may be directly visualised.

It is well to remember that when the blood pressure is recorded in the standard fashion account is taken of the girth of the upper arm for the greater the girth the higher has to be the pressure in the inflated cuff to occlude the underlying artery and so the higher the apparent blood pressure. The objectives of investigation of hypertensive patients are firstly to define more accurately the degree of damage to the heart and kidneys in particular and secondly to look for a possible underlying cause. All patients therefore should be submitted to a chemical and microscopic urine analysis, urine culture, estimation of blood urea and electrolytes, endogenous creatinine clearance, E.C.G. and chest X-ray procedures. If there are sufficient clinical suspicions or on the basis of the results of these screening investigations, further, more sophisticated investigations may be required to search for a primary cause, such as urine collections for adrenal hormone assays, intravenous pyelography, isotope renography and aortography. If a primary cause is found it will require appropriate treatment. However the very nature of most of the kidney diseases which may give rise to hypertension, precludes cure and the majority of these are managed in the same way as the situation of essential hypertension for which no cause has been found. Obese patients should be advised to lose weight and this measure alone may be sufficient to restore the blood pressure to normal if it is only mildly elevated. If the patient is psychoneurotic the use of sedatives or tranquilizers may prove helpful. For patients unresponsive to these procedures a thiazide diuretic may be effective, apparently because of an effect on small blood vessels. In some severe instances these measures may be insufficient and the use of an antihypertensive drug will be required. The dose of these has to be adjusted to maintain normal or near normal levels of blood pressure. Most patients respond adequately to this form of management and the blood pressure can be kept under control often for many years. A few unfortunate individuals have very high blood pressure which cannot be properly reduced and which is quickly complicated by damage to the brain, heart and kidneys. This is the situation of malignant hypertension which usually despite all therapeutic efforts, ends fatally in some six months to two years. Organ damage in the course of the benign form of the disease may likewise shorten the patient's life expectancy.

Left Heart Failure.

Often a dramatic event this occurrence may be the result of left atrial or left ventricular failure in the first instance. The end result of both is pulmonary oedema because of accumulation of blood in the lungs. Mitral stenosis is by far the commonest cause of left atrial failure while left ventricular failure may be due to mitral incompetence, aortic valve disease, systemic hypertension or some other less common situations. There is usually severe breathlessness of sudden onset, accompanied by cyanosis and expectoration of pink frothy sputum. Affected patients are gravely ill and require emergency management. The underlying cause, such as valvular heart disease may be confirmed on examination of the heart and auscultation of the lungs will reveal the presence of the widespread fine crepitations characteristic of pulmonary oedema. Many patients have developed left ventricular failure as a result of a myocardial infarction, but because of the clamant feature of breathlessness they may have appreciated little or no chest pain. Appropriate investigations should be instituted to look for this possibility while a chest X-ray commonly confirms the pattern of pulmonary oedema. As intimated treatment must be implemented without delay, oxygen should be administered continuously and the doctor will usually give morphine, digoxin, aminophylline and frusemide by the intravenous route. Rapid improvement thereafter is often very striking, the patient having been literally returned from the brink of death. Digoxin and diuretic therapy must thereafter be continued as required to effect complete control of the heart failure. When the patient's condition has been stabilised in this way attention can then be given to the precipitating cause and management appropriately instituted. There is a high mortality rate from left heart failure, a notable proportion of patients succumbing before they reach hospital. Even when the crisis has been overcome the severity of the underlying disease often leads to a poor eventual outcome.

Congestive Cardiac Failure.

By common usage this term is restricted to the description of the clinical features which accompany failure of the right side of the heart. Although it may occur in an acute form, especially in association with massive pulmonary embolism, the condition is more commonly of a chronic nature and is most frequently associated with chronic lung disease (which may be due to long standing left sided heart disease such as mitral stenosis) or myocardial ischaemia. Patients with chronic congestive cardiac failure frequently present with the complaint of ankle swelling often accompanied by undue exertional dyspnoea and fatigue. They may in addition experience diminished appetite, nausea and even abdominal pain and vomiting from congestion of the abdominal organs. The outstanding physical findings are related to the accumulation of fluid which results from relative stagnation of the circulation. Thus ankle oedema, sacral oedema and over distension of the neck veins are virtually invariable findings. Less commonly the liver may be engorged and tender and there may be ascites. Examination of the heart and lungs usually reveals the nature of the underlying disease which may be confirmed by E.C.G. and Chest X-ray procedures. A significant proportion of patients with borderline cardiac failure are precipitated into frank failure by a superimposed chest infection. Sputum culture in this situation is therefore desirable. Bed rest is essential and a low salt diet with fluid restriction is usually imposed. Diuretic therapy and digitalisation are employed to clear the fluid overload and to restore the cardiac output to nearer normal values. Appropriate antibiotic therapy will be necessary if active chest infection is present. The patients are usually more comfortable if they are propped up in bed. Careful records of fluid balance should be kept and the patient weighed regularly to assess the efficacy of therapy in promoting a diuresis and reducing the volume of excess tissue fluid which has accumulated. In most instances initial therapy is successful and usually maintenance treatment with diuretics and digoxin has to be continued to reduce the likelihood of relapse. The eventual outcome is largely determined by the nature of the underlying disease.

Deep Venous Thrombosis.

In itself rarely a serious condition, the main danger of deep venous thrombosis lies in its potential to be complicated by the often grave situation of pulmonary embolism. While there are numerous factors which are known to predispose to thrombosis in the large veins of the lower limbs and pelvis, the commonest and most important are pregnancy and prolonged immobility, particularly after surgical operation and in association with infections and dehydration. Use of the contraceptive pill is becoming a progressively more frequent cause. In all too many patients the presence of a venous thrombosis is only suspected after an episode of pulmonary embolism occurs, for in such patients there are no abnormal physical signs in the lower limbs. When clinical features are present they are often of sudden onset with pain in the calf followed by swelling of the leg. In the full blown case the leg is symmetrically swollen, flushed and hot. The superficial veins may be dilated and pitting oedema is often demonstrable. Tenderness is usually maximal in the calf over the site of the deep veins. Such a clinical picture is unmistakable but in less obvious instances it may be advisable to obtain confirmation of venous occlusion by venography (a technique similar to arteriography), if this facility is available. Management of the acute phase must be rigorously supervised to minimise the risk of potentially fatal complications. Complete bed rest is essential, a bed cage should be provided and the end of the bed should be elevated. These manoeuvres facilitate resolution of oedema and stabilisation of the thrombus. Anticoagulant therapy initially as a continuous intravenous infusion of heparin should be started, (in the absence of frank contra-indications such as an established duodenal ulcer) and continued by oral drugs for a period of six months. When pain has subsided and swelling and tenderness have virtually resolved cautious mobilisation may be initiated. These features do not normally become apparent until a period of one to two weeks has elapsed. Provided that the problem of pulmonary embolism can be avoided (and there is no guarantee in the individual that it can) the prognosis is for most patients excellent although some residual discomfort and swelling may persist.

Peripheral Arterial Disease.

Restricting the term to describe a disease of the arteries supplying the limbs, particularly the lower limbs, resulting from their progressive narrowing, this condition bears striking similarities to coronary artery disease. In both the presence of plaques of material known as atheroma can be visualised within the affected vessels. Again it seems that in this disease as it affects the limbs smoking and dietary factors play important roles. The disease is more common in patients who have diabetes mellitus and in them complications such as cellulitis are more frequently encountered. As in coronary artery disease pain is often experienced in the ischaemic part. In the limbs this is known as claudication and is more readily experienced on exercise and exposure to cold. With progression in the severity of the disease pain may even occur at rest, characteristically in bed, when the unduly warm environment demands an increased blood supply to the exposed lower limbs. Ischaemic skin is unduly sensitive to even the slightest damage and highly prone to infection. These factors serve to complicate the problem of management further. Complete occlusion of vessels may result in actual gangrene of the affected part. The skin of a limb which has a poor blood supply is often thin, inelastic, cold, hairless and of impaired sensitivity. Arterial pulses may be poor in volume or even absent. Discolouration and absence of sensation in an area is an ominous sign suggestive of incipient gangrene. All patients with peripheral arterial disease should be screened for diabetes mellitus. Arteriography may be useful to define the extent and severity of the lesions, particularly if surgery is contemplated. Mildly affected patients should be advised to give up smoking and to limit but not to give up exercise. Skin of the involved limbs must be protected by suitable footwear and careful attention to chiropody should be given since many complications have arisen from damage done while cutting the toe-nails. Some patients will be candidates for reconstructive surgery. When gangrene supervenes all attempts must be made to prevent or eradicate infection with suitable dressings and antibiotic therapy. Diabetes mellitus if present will require separate management. Once gangrene has become established the prognosis is largely dependent on the degree to which it localises and to what extent the involved limb is amenable to surgery.

11
Diseases of the Nervous System

Epilepsy.

Encompassing a wide variety of neurological disorders characterised by abnormal electrical activity in the brain and often manifest as involuntary movements, this group of conditions may stem from numerous causes. On some instances it appears that from birth certain brain cells are destined to function improperly. Other cases of epilepsy appear to originate from structural brain disease such as occurs in cerebral tumours or after head injuries, while a number of patients suffer seizures which seem to result from metabolic upsets like hypoxia, hypoglycaemia and uraemia. The commonest form of epilepsy is the 'grand mal' type which classically has four distinct phases. Preceding the appearance of the involuntary movements there is frequently an aura which is a sensation commonly similar to that perceived by one of the special senses. Hence the patient may appreciate odd visual phenomena or smells, and he soon comes to associate these with an impending fit. There then follows the tonic convulsion, during which there is loss of consciousness with generalised limb and trunk rigidity, clenching of teeth and often biting of the tongue. At this stage there is often involuntary emptying of the bladder or bowel. This phase soon gives way to one of clonic seizures when convulsive movements occur in rapid succession. These may continue for several minutes or even longer and are then usually replaced by the final phase of relaxation, gradual return of consciousness and eventual recovery. Occasionally grand mal seizures persist without relenting, giving rise to the condition of status epilepticus, which not infrequently ends in death from exhaustion. Other forms of epilepsy, such as the petit mal, Jacksonian and temporal lobe types are distinctly less common. Investigation of epileptic patients often involves highly sophisticated techniques but such procedures as plain X-ray of skull and electro-encephalography are usually available. Treatment for grand mal epilepsy can be considered at two separate levels. Firstly there is the management of the actual fit and secondly the consideration of treatment aimed at prevention of further seizures. When a fit occurs attempts should be made to insert a gag into the patient's mouth to minimise damage to the tongue. Movements should not otherwise be restrained but the surrounding area should, as far as possible be cleared of objects upon which the patient may injure himself. If anti-convulsant drugs are available they should be adminstered as quickly as possible, given intra-muscularly or if technically feasible may be given intravenously. When the convulsions have been controlled in this way the patient is then allowed to rest and regain consciousness. It will then frequently be necessary to continue treatment by the oral route to prevent recurrences – the actual dose being determined by the clinical response. A number of patients whose epilepsy is congenital appear to improve as they grow older and in some anti-convulsant therapy may be discontinued. Others suffer isolated attacks for example associated with an episode of hypoglycaemia which do not recur and hence no further treatment is required, while an unfortunate significant proportion of patients continue to endure seizures from time to time despite all attempts to suppress them.

Parkinsonism.

A syndrome resulting from localised damage to the brain, most commonly due to arterial disease, this condition is nowadays largely restricted to the middle-aged and elderly. The main symptom is usually that of tremor, particularly of the hands. In addition there is often a degree of rigidity of the limbs, tremor of the lips and in more advanced cases over-production of saliva, monotony of speech, lack of facial expression and difficulty in walking. The clinical features are in most instances of gradual onset and slow progression, though some patients are eventually incapacitated by the disorder. Tremor is the outstanding sign in the majority of patients and may be abolished by conscious effort. Rigidity is of rather a different form than that encountered in the stroke patients. The mask-like face, shuffling gait and other features are less commonly encountered. The diagnosis is based entirely on clinical appraisal. Management rests largely on regular physiotherapy to maintain the residual useful motor function, especially in the limbs, and the use of atropine-like drugs such as Benzhexol. A few patients are suitable candidates for specialised brain surgery which may be dramatically effective, but the most the majority of patients can hope for is arrest or limitation of the progression of their disease by conservative measures. In the great majority of patients there is little restriction of overall activity.

Disseminated Sclerosis.

A disease prevalent in young, otherwise healthy adults, the cause of this condition is as yet undetermined though the end result is patchy loss of the covering sheath of nerve fibres in the central nervous system with subsequent loss of their function. Symptoms and signs are extremely varied in nature and severity which makes early diagnosis often extremely difficult. Sudden onset of double vision or loss of sight is a characteristic presenting complaint and is particularly suggestive of disseminated sclerosis when recovery occurs spontaneously. Often, however, initial symptoms are less outstanding such as loss of sensation over a small area of skin or transient limb weakness. Classically the disease follows a course of relapse and remission with progressively increasing incapacity with each episode. Eventually affected individuals, after a period of some years, become bed-ridden, or confined to a wheelchair and many experience considerable difficulty with bladder and bowel control. The phases of relapse remit without treatment, in many instances. The distribution of the apparent nerve lesions seems quite haphazard in the full blown case so that the abnormal vision and eye movements, tremors, loss of sensation, weakness and staggering are commonly identifiable. Some patients are noted to be rather carefree in their attitude to their disabilities and this may represent a further manifestation of their disease. In view of the difficulty frequently experienced in reaching any definite clinical conclusions it is well to be guarded in expressing an opinion on the nature of the disease until there have been further opportunities to observe the patient's progress. Various tests on the cerebro-spinal fluid may be helpful but are by no means conclusive. Treatment is essentially based on persistent physiotherapy to ensure the maximum use of remaining muscle function. Some patients seem to gain short-term benefit from a course of injections of A.C.T.H. The outlook is bleak for most patients, with an increased susceptibility to infection accounting in many instances for eventual death.

Cerebro-vascular Accidents.

These phenomena include extradural and subdural haemorrhage

which are usually due to trauma and are hence the province of the surgeon. The physician encounters spontaneous subarachnoid haemorrhage and intracerebral thrombosis, embolism and haemorrhage, commonly in medical wards. Spontaneous subarachnoid haemorrhage results from rupture of an arterial aneurysm at the base of the brain or bleeding from an intracranial tumour. Classically there is sudden onset of severe headache which characteristically radiates from the back of the head to the front and is associated with vomiting and often loss of consciousness. Some patients may have experienced several preceding similar episodes. Stiffness of the neck and impairment of consciousness are common findings and a significant number of the patients are hypertensive. When the episode has been severe there may be diminished or absent pupillary reflexes and visible oedema or haemorrhage in the fundus of the eye. Frequently there are no other notable findings though some patients suffer paralysis and sensory loss. If the patient survives, all efforts should be made to determine the cause of the bleeding, for the lesion if discovered may be amenable to surgery correction and hence recurrences may be prevented. Unless contra-indicated (by the presence of oedema in the optic fundi) lumbar puncture should be performed. If this is done soon after the episode has occurred, fresh blood is usually demonstrable in the cerebro-spinal fluid and the diagnosis thereby confirmed. X-rays of skull and arteriography of the cerebral circulation are required to aid identification of the underlying abnormality. It is generally recommended that a patient should be confined to bed for some six weeks after such an episode in an effort to minimise the risk of recurrence. When it is technically feasible and clinically desirable to correct the basic defect surgically, this is usually advised. Many patients die quickly as a result of the haemorrhage. The outlook for survivors is improved if they are candidates for surgery. Of those who are not, many succumb to a second haemorrhage often occurring within six months of the first episode.

Intracerebral thrombosis, embolism and haemorrhage tend to produce the clinical syndrome known as a 'stroke', since they regularly affect the same area of one or other half of the brain. As a result the patient experiences usually sudden loss of power in the arm and leg of one side and in the corresponding side of the face. Because of the anatomical relationship of nerve fibres in the brain a cerebro-vascular accident in one half produces paralysis of the opposite side of the body. If the right side of the body is affected speech is commonly disturbed in addition. Many of these patients have arteriosclerotic disease of the cerebral blood vessels and many are hypertensive. In contrast most of those who have suffered a cerebral embolism (and in whom a site of extra-cranial thrombosis can be shown, as in mitral stenosis) are in a younger age group. Distinction between thrombosis and haemorrhage in the individual patient during life is frequently impossible: severely affected patients rapidly lose consciousness and in this group many die quickly. Others survive to suffer a variable degree of hemiparesis and speech defect. In addition to loss of power, spasticity poses a major problem in mobilisation and re-education of limbs. Bladder and bowel control is often also disordered. Those patients who have at the worst only slight disability may benefit greatly from speech and physiotherapy. Where more severe deficiencies exist the prospect of useful recovery is less likely and it is these patients who require long-term care and impose considerable loads on the nursing services. If the episode of 'stroke' can be established as being caused by cerebral embolism it is often advisable to embark on long term anticoagulant therapy in the hope of preventing a recurrence. The inadvertent or ill advised use of anticoagulants in cerebral thrombosis and haemorrhage can of course be disastrous as a result of intra cerebral bleeding. The various procedures involved in the care of the unconscious patient are laid out in Section II.

Peripheral Neuropathy.

An ever increasing number of agents have been implicated as causing damage to peripheral nerves. Infections such as diphtheria, metabolic disorders e.g. diabetes mellitus, poisoning as with lead, deficiency states like pernicious anaemia and chronic alcoholism are only a few of the disorders which are known to produce the clinical picture of peripheral neuropathy. One, a few or many nerves may be affected and the damage may be permanent or reversible according to the cause. Symptoms are usually of paraesthesiae (tingling and 'pins and needles') and weakness in the affected parts. If the disorder is widespread there may be life threatening complications such as paralysis of the respiratory muscles. Testing the various forms of sensation often reveals loss or diminished appreciation of stimuli, while tone and motor power are usually reduced, and reflexes absent. Wasting of involved muscles may be striking if the disease has been established for some time. There is usually a diagnostic lead from the patient's history to help decide the precise cause and hence allow appropriate treatment. Investigations are often required however to confirm the diagnosis and their nature is determined by the probabilities suggested by the clinical features. Treatment must of course be directed at the underlying conditions and in addition physio-therapeutic manoevres should be utilised to maintain residual power and tone while hopefully awaiting spontaneous restoration of nerve function or improvement as a result of correction of the underlying disorder.

Section II

The nurse can help greatly by understanding and by giving time to talk with the patient but where possible the Medical Social Worker is the most suitable person to cope with this situation. She has liaison with other groups outwith the hospital and can be of considerable support to the patient and his family during the "crisis."

Patients who are physically or mentally handicapped have very specific problems with which the nurse must be able to cope. The blind patient is a very typical example of where forethought is essential. The patient is unable to see what is going on around him but is usually very perceptive to atmosphere. It is important for the nurse to speak as she approaches the bed. Explanation of a procedure prior to doing it and also during it gives the patient confidence and allows for maximum co-operation.

The deaf patient may or may not have a hearing aid, but if it is difficult to communicate by speech then the nurse must take time to convey to the patient her intentions, by using signs. If the patient has a hearing aid, ensure it is in working order and he is encouraged to wear it while in the ward.

The careful handling of artificial limbs is another of the nurse's responsibilities. To the patient these things are of vast importance and it is essential that the nurse lets the patient see that they are safely stored until the time comes for them to be used again.

Dentures are also important to the patient — and whenever possible these should be worn. If however they are not then again the patient must know that they are safely in store until they are in use again.

This book has covered nursing care in relation to specific diseases but there is much more than nursing care when one considers total patient care. The patient as a whole must be considered and not only the disease which caused his admission. Some patients have been considered in the previous paragraphs, there are many more and as a nurse one must consider all aspects concerned with total patient care.

In addition to all the theoretical training and education you have had remember the old fashioned qualification called "common sense"; the height of the seat of a chair, the tiring troublesome visitor, a sympathetic ear, a kindly touch, altering the light shining on the

Section II

The various procedures relevant to the management of patients in medical wards, at which the nurse will be expected to become proficient, are described and their nature and application explained.

This text is designed to be used in conjunction with the systematic lectures which will cover the subjects discussed. For the purposes of reference larger and more specialised text books should be consulted.

Patient Care

There are always patients in the ward who have a need for a different approach by the nurse. She has to develop an understanding of people and remember each patient is an individual whose reactions to hospital can vary considerably. Much of this understanding comes from experience but some of it can be learned by giving thought to each situation as it arises.

There is the patient who is very withdrawn, he does not appear to talk with the other patients and seems to make very little effort to help himself. On the other hand one will have the patient who talks incessantly and wants to know about everything that is happening. Two extremes, but how often one finds this situation in the ward. A different approach is required for each of these patients because temperamentally they are different but basically one must consider that they are both worried by being in hospital and are reacting in different ways.

Now consider other situations, e.g. those which can give rise to the patient feeling "depressed." The mother who has a young family at home dependent on relations or neighbours looking after them. The husband who may lose his job as a result of being off work for some time. The elderly couple separated as a result of one of them being in hospital and the other maybe not able to cope with being alone.

patient's face, wilting flowers, coping with the unsuitable gift from visitors, clean fresh appearance — no textbook can teach you about these and many similar situations in day-to-day nursing. This is just what nursing is about coupled with sound and practical theoretical knowledge.

E.L.

General Nursing Duties

Before considering the specialised nursing techniques required for individual illnesses or for the nursing part in the special Diagnostic Technique Section there are several general and important nursing duties which are essential in the correct and accurate assessment of the patient's illness.

Nurse must always remember that but for her constant, careful, and accurate vigilance the doctor's assessment of the patient's progress would be impossible.

Fluid Balance Charts

Fluid balance charts are important, but in order to be useful they must be accurate. All urine should be measured even when a bowel movement has occured at the same time.

Fluid intake must also be accurately assessed. This is always more difficult but there are two ways of ensuring its success — either giving the patient a measured amount of fluid when required or the patient may be given a jug containing a measured amount of water and the amount taken by the patient entered in the fluid chart each time the jug is changed, e.g. if a jug which contains 500 mls when changed contains 200 mls the amount taken by the patient is 300 mls.

There are times when fluid intake must be restricted and this is when accurate charts are invaluable in assessing progress because the purpose of restricting intake is usually to encourage absorption and excretion of excess tissue fluid.

MIDNIGHT — MIDNIGHT
INTAKE & OUTPUT CHART

	INTAKE		TIME	OUTPUT		NOTES
	Details	Amount		Details	Amount	
JUG CHANGED	WATER (500ml)	—	Midnight			
			1			
			2			
			3			
			4	URINE	300mls	
			5			
			6			
	TEA: MILK	300mls	7	URINE	100mls	
JUG CHANGED	WATER (500ml)	300mls	8			
			9			
	MID-MORNING DRINK	180mls	10			
			11	URINE	360mls	+ BOWEL MOVEMENT.
	SOUP: MILK	360mls	Noon			
			1			
JUG CHANGED	WATER (500ml)	250mls	2	URINE	200mls	
			3			
	TEA	180mls	4			
			5			
	TEA	180mls	6	URINE	360mls	
JUG CHANGED	WATER (500)	200mls	7			
			8			
	EVENING DRINK	180mls	9			
			10	URINE	350mls	
			11			
	WATER	250mls	Midnight			
	Total Intake	2380mls		Total Output	1660mls.	

Of course the purpose of fluid balance charts does not stop at intake of fluid by mouth, and output of urine. They are a means of recording the amount of fluid given intravenously and the amount of fluid loss from the body by way of chest aspiration, haematemesis, melaena,

MIDNIGHT — MIDNIGHT
INTAKE & OUTPUT CHART

INTAKE			TIME	OUTPUT		NOTES
Details	IV	Amount ORAL		Details	Amount	
NORMAL SALINE	500		Midnight			
			1	URINE	200mls	
			2			
			3	VOMITUS	200mls	BILE STAINED
MILK		100	4			
			5			
5% DEXTROSE	500		6			
MILK		100	7	URINE	300mls	+ BOWEL MOVEMENT
			8			(MELAENA)
			9			
WEAK TEA		100	10			
			11			
5% DEXTROSE	500		Noon	URINE	250 mls	
			1			
			2			
MILK		100	3			
			4	VOMITUS	100 mls	+VE. BLOOD
			5			
NORMAL SALINE	250 500		6			AMOUNT OF N/SALINE DISCARDED 1.250mls
MILK		100	7	VOMITUS	250 mls	+VE BLOOD.
BLOOD	500		8			BLOOD No. 1763
			9			
			10	URINE	300 mls	
			11			MN. - TO START NEW UNIT OF BLOOD
BLOOD			Midnight			TOTAL CARRIED
Total Intake	2250 mls	500 mls		Total Output	1600mls	FORWARD TO NEXT CHART

Form No. 147

and vomitus, to mention but a few routes.

Accurate recording and reporting of blood loss and fluid loss such as in vomiting, will be vital to the patient's recovery if replacement therapy is necessary.

Intravenous Fluids and Blood

Although the starting of an infusion is not the nurse's responsibility she is responsible for observing the patient while he is receiving the infusion. Observation does not only mean watching that the bottle does not completely empty before changing it, but noting the patient's reaction to the infusion and reporting any change in his condition to the medical staff.

The time within which an infusion is to run, is determined by the physician in charge, and the rate of flow can be calculated from this.

Some physicians may regulate the rate of flow, but this does not always happen and the nurse must therefore be able to perform this task.

The most frequently used intravenous fluids are in bottles containing approximately 540 mls.

If the bottle has to run in over 12 hours — $\frac{540}{12}$	= 45 mls/hour
$\frac{45}{60}$	= 0.75 mls/minute
There are 15 minims — drops ml. $\therefore$	= 11 drops/minute.
Over 8 hours — using the above mentioned method of calculation,	= 17 drops/minute
Over 4 hours —	= 33 drops/minute

There are occasions when blood presented in the form of packed cells or blood derivitives such as plasma may be made up in units of 300 mls. Under these circumstances the above calculations would be adapted to suit this amount.

To prepare for setting up an infusion, one requires on the lower shelf of a trolley:

1. pack containing sterile swabs
2. cotton wool balls
3. gallipot and drapes
4. skin cleansing agent
5. various intravenous cannulae
6. arm splint
7. adhesive or micropore tape
8. bandage
9. infusion set

The top shelf of the trolley will be prepared to receive the sterile articles and a disposal bag will be attached to the side of the trolley.

To prepare the infusion set ready for use, it is advisable to prime it with normal saline solution, which is isotonic to blood and will, to some extent, help to prevent clotting at the tip of the needle when first inserted into the vein. To do this quickly, move the control clamp up the tubing, to within 9 — 12 cm of the lower chamber and fasten tightly. Insert the needle and airway, if it is a separate item, into the bottle and apply gentle pressure to the sides of the upper chamber. This will fill with fluid. The lower chamber will also fill but no fluid will enter the tubing. When both chambers are filled to approximately 2 cm, slowly release the clamp and allow the tubing to fill expelling all air. The set is now ready for use.

Observation of the patient has already been mentioned as being of importance, but there are other points which must be stressed:—

1. *Blood*

Never have blood lying in the ward unless it is going to be used immediately or within a very short time.

Always have the label on the bottle or pack checked by another member of staff — preferably a senior member — when it is to be put up. This should be done at the bedside, where one can check: name, address and date of birth, with the patient, if he is able, or with the patient's bed card.

To complete the transfusion it is advisable to run through some normal saline so that the patient receives the full amount of blood.

Some patients may show signs of adverse reaction to the blood. Symptoms include, sudden elevation in temperature, rapid pulse, dyspnoea, pain in chest and anuria. Medical advice must always be sought when such circumstances arise.

2. *Fluids*

When a patient is to receive fluid intravenously, the physician will define the regime he wishes followed and the time over which each bottle has to run. This is usually quite straightforward, but there are circumstances when it is necessary to add other substances to the bottles. This is done by the medical staff. There is now the responsibility of ensuring that the right patient receives the correct bottle. One must therefore carry out the routine of checking as for blood.

When the infusion is complete or has to be discontinued for any reason it will probably be the nurse's responsibility to remove the needle from the vein. To do this

1. turn the control clamp off
2. remove all strapping
3. place a sterile swab over the needle at it's point of insertion through the skin
4. apply firm pressure over the swab
5. with the other hand pull the needle out
6. maintain pressure over the site for a few minutes to prevent the formation of a haematoma and apply a firm sterile dressing

As the patient will be confined to bed during an infusion, good general nursing care is important such as oral hygiene, attention to pressure areas, assistance with washing and toilet care, but there is one point which must not be forgotten. The patient may be able to feed himself but it is impossible to cut up food when one arm is immobilised. It is therefore important to perform this task for the patient.

One further point — never tamper with infusions. If it is not running, by all means remove the bandage, it may be too firmly applied, but if this measure does not give rise to improvement the medical staff must be informed.

Naso-Gastric Feeding

There are occasions when the patient is unable to take solids or fluids by mouth in sufficient quantity to maintain a normal nutritional balance essential to life and therefore his nourishment must be given by some other route. There are two ways by which food can be put directly into the stomach other than by eating.

1 by gastrostomy tube
2 by naso-gastric tube

It is the latter which is more likely to be encountered in medical nursing. (See Page 82).

Requirements:

(a) To pass tube —

naso-gastric tube	lubricant
swabs	drapes
litmus or pH. paper	spigot
sickness bowl	50 ml. syringe with catheter tip

(b) For feeding —

tray on which there is a jug containing the measured feed at the correct temperature.

bowl with hot water in which to sit the jug during feeding in order to keep the feed at a suitable temperature.

The patient is usually more able to co-operate in the initial stages of passing the tube over the back of the throat if he is lying in a semi-recumbent position. It is most important to explain the procedure in detail to the patient before starting because it is an uncomfortable experience and can be quite frightening, but a nurse who is confident in her approach and proficient in carrying out the procedure, can go a long way in allaying fear and apprehension in a patient.

If the patient is unconscious, the medical staff will pass the tube. There are great risks to passing a tube when the patient is unable to co-operate, principally due to the possible absence of cough and swallowing reflexes, this could result in the tube passing into the trachea and bronchi, with serious consequences.

To pass the tube

Lubricate the tube for approximately three inches from the tip. Hold it between the thumb and index finger and pass it over the back of the tongue to the throat. Instruct your patient to breath through his mouth during this stage of the procedure. When the tip of the tube touches the back of the throat ask your patient to swallow, this reflex movement will take the tube over the pharynx into the oesophagus. Continue to pass the tube slowly, ask the patient to swallow each time the tube is moved. When the desired length of tube has been passed it is very important to check its position before a feed is given. The tube can be passed into the stomach by way of the nose rather than the mouth. The nostrils must be quite clear, the lubricated end of the tube is passed very gently along the floor of the nose until it passes into the naso-pharynx from which point the procedure is as above. Attach a syringe to the tube and aspirate, if no fluid is obtained alter the position of the tube and again aspirate. When fluid is obtained it must be tested with pH. paper to determine the presence of acid indicating the tube is in position.

The position of the tube can be checked by one other method other than X-ray. A syringe containing 20 mls. air is attached to the tube. Listen with a stethoscope over the area of the stomach, slowly inject the air down the tube and it will be heard entering the stomach.

The Size of Feed

The size of feed is important as it is hoped to avoid vomiting or regurgitation of fluid. Approximately 300 mls. given every 3 hours, will give an adequate fluid intake over a 24 hour period. Calorie value will, of course, depend on the type of feed given.

Method (1)

Using a 50 ml. syringe with catheter tip is ideal. The piston is removed. It is easily cleaned and is disposable and a fresh one can be used each day. It can be attached directly to the naso-gastric tube and the rate of flow can be easily controlled without using a clamp.

Method (2)

Using the "drip" method — An intravenous infusion bottle filled with the amount of feed to be given. An infusion set with the cannula connection cut off, a portex connection suitable in size to fit the end of the naso-gastric tube on one side and the infusion set on the other side. The infusion set is filled with the feed before it is connected to the naso-gastric tube. The rate of flow is controlled by the clamp on the tubing.

Although nursing time is not being used in the "drip" method observation of the patient must be made frequently in order to detect early signs of intolerance of the feed.

Collection of 24 Hour Specimen of Urine

Usually the most convenient time to start a collection is in the morning when the patient first rises. At this time he is asked to pass urine which is discarded, the time is noted and the collection is continued until the same hour the next day, all urine passed during this time being put into the specific container clearly marked with the patient's name and ward number. There are many reasons for collecting urine specimens and there are different containers in use for this purpose some of which have in them a preservative. It is therefore important to ensure that the correct container is used as this saves time both at ward and laboratory level. There are some specimens which require to have blood sent with them, e.g. creatinine clearance. It is important therefore to check on this point.

If the patient is up and about in the ward he can be instructed in the management of his collection, but if he is on bed rest it is wise to tell him that he is "on a collection" and that if he is to have a bowel movement to use, if possible, a separate bedpan for this purpose.

Collection of a Midstream Specimen of Urine

This is an uncontaminated specimen of urine obtained without catheterisation, and the preparation of the patient must be meticulous. As it is an aseptic technique it is necessary to prepare a trolley in advance so that it can be taken to the bedside when the patient is ready to pass urine. This procedure requires the co-operation of the patient.

Female Patient

The patient should lie in a reclining position with a bedpan under the buttocks. Using sterile water swab the outer vaginal area, one swab for each side, separate the labia and again swab both sides using a fresh swab for each side, and finally swab over the urethra. Swabbing of the genital area is not always essential, thorough washing and drying is equally effective prior to collecting the specimen.

Ask the patient to pass a little urine and then stop, place the sterile receptacle in position below the patient and ask her to pass urine into it. When there is enough urine for a specimen withdraw the container and leave the patient to complete emptying her bladder. Transfer the specimen to a sterile bottle to send to the laboratory.

Male Patient

If the patient has been circumcised the urethral opening and immediately surrounding area are swabbed and the collection made in a manner similar to that for the female patient. If the patient has not been circumcised the foreskin should be retracted sufficiently to expose the urethral opening and held in this position during the remainder of the procedure. The majority of male patients can satisfactorily carry out the whole manoeuvre without assistance.

Care of the Dying

Nurses are closely concerned with all aspects of patient care and that which is most demanding, emotionally, is the care of the patient who is dying. Reaction to this situation is highly individual and often the younger the nurse is, the greater is the emotional effect.

There are many times when the nurse/patient relationship is very close, and should the death of the patient occur the effect can be very upsetting to the nurse concerned. There is no shame in private feelings.

Care of the dying must be allied to care of the living, especially the relatives, because it is they who really need the greatest support and comfort. Consideration must be given to their wish to be with the patient as much as possible during this period. One will find they are only too willing to be of assistance e.g. with feeding or drinks for the patient, and they feel that they are being useful to the nurse in the ward, but this does not remove her main responsibility, that is, giving continuous good nursing care. If relatives are with the patient never delay giving the attention necessary, they will be only too pleased to be displaced for a short time and, if possible, a cup of tea should be made available.

Unfortunately there are occasions when a patient will die alone. This situation may not be avoidable and feelings of guilt on the part of the nurse are natural but in almost every instance they are ill-founded as other duties have usually demanded attention at the time.

In the ward other patients are very often aware of a death and have the normal reaction to this situation, but the daily routine should take up its usual pattern within a very short time.

There are many opinions as to the most satisfactory position for the dying patient's bed in the ward.

1. *The Unconscious Patient*

The patient in this state requires very intensive nursing care and should be so positioned in the ward that this can be done frequently and also so that he can be kept under constant surveillance.

2. *The Conscious Patient Showing Signs of Deterioration*

If he remains alert and comfortable, it is often wise to leave him among those with whom he has become familiar until his condition is causing distress to the others around him. At this point moving him to the acute nursing area is often advisable.

Relatives' reaction is unpredictable at the time of death of a loved one, no matter how long or short the terminal stage has been, the grief can be great. The relatives may wish to see the deceased before they leave, and the nurse should be prepared for this. The bed must be screened. The body will be dressed ready for the mortuary, and the bedclothes so arranged over it that the deceased appears to be sleeping. Flowers should be placed on the locker and chairs placed at the side of the bed. The relatives are escorted in and left alone for a few minutes with the deceased.

When transferred to the mortuary, as an act of courtesy, one should escort the body for a short distance out of the ward.

Nursing Care in Congestive Cardiac Failure

On admission the patient is sometimes very distressed and apprehensive and hence requires much reassurance. There is occasionally marked dyspnoea even at rest due to pulmonary oedema, and a varying degree of generalised oedema and cyanosis is often apparent.

The nurse's most important aim is to make the patient as comfortable as possible in bed. This can be achieved by arranging the pillows in arm-chair fashion so that they give adequate support and keep the patient in an upright position. Bedclothes should be light and a bedcage in position will prevent them causing pressure on the lower limbs. Often a patient will feel more comfortable if he can lean forward on a firm surface e.g. a bedtable with a pillow on top. This position fixes the shoulder girdle and enables the accessory muscles of respiration to come into use, so that dyspnoea is often relieved or becomes more easily tolerated.

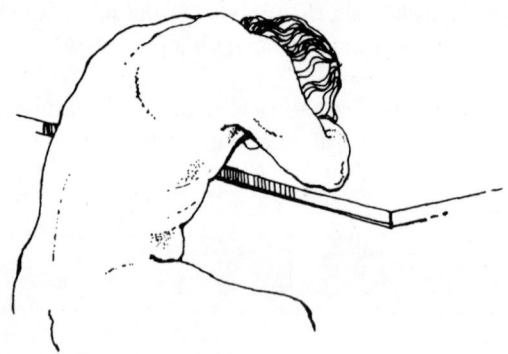

Recording temperature, pulse and respiration, and noting in particular pulse rate and rhythm and reporting any abnormality is of considerable importance when digoxin is being given to improve cardiac output, as one of the earliest signs of digoxin overdosage is coupling of the beats. If oxygen is ordered, ensure that the correct rate of flow is registering on the flowmeter, that the humidifier is filled to the correct level, and that the mask is the correct type, fitting well, and is comfortable.

The patient is usually given a diuretic to increase urinary output, so charting of fluid intake and output must be accurate. If the patient is grossly oedematous and urine output is poor, even with a diuretic, fluid intake may require to be restricted to e.g. 500–1000 mls. This volume will require to be given in divided amounts over the whole 24 hours period, as one usually finds that a patient with this condition does not sleep throughout the night but for short periods during the 24 hours. The reasons for restricting fluids must be explained to the patient in order to have his co-operation. There is no sense in allowing the patient to take fluids freely, although his output may be as much as, or a little greater than, his intake, since the problem of fluid retention within the tissues is not being solved. Restriction in fluid causes a greater absorption of the excess fluid from within the tissues and the diuretic is effective by its power to stimulate the excretion of this fluid in the form of urine. Finally, the patient must be encouraged to expectorate as this will improve ventilation of the lung tissue and oxygenation of the blood.

There are times when the patient may feel more comfortable and at ease if permitted to sit in a chair for long periods rather than in bed. In this position breathing is easier and he feels less dependent on assistance with feeding and toilet. However this should only be attempted after consultation with the physician in charge of the patient's care.

If the patient is unfit to get out of bed, good basic nursing care is essential to his comfort and wellbeing. Care and attention to pressure areas, and especially when oedema is present frequent change of position is essential. Encourage the patient to move his lower limbs while in bed as this prevents stasis of the circulation and the development of a deep vein thrombosis. Oral hygiene is especially important when the patient is on restricted fluids. Diet is also of importance — the physician may consider the patient would benefit from one which is salt free or has no added salt especially when the patient is oedematous.

When mobilisation commences this is done slowly, half an hour the first day, an hour the second day, increasing the time out of bed by a little more each day. While the patient is up sitting in a chair, a footstool must always be available on which to keep his legs elevated to prevent the natural gravitation of oedema to ankles and feet as would occur in the normal sitting position. When he is oedema free and more mobile this will not be necessary.

Nursing Care in Left Ventricular Failure

In this condition the patient suffers from acute attacks of dyspnoea, which can occur either on exertion, or during the night when he is lying in bed asleep. In the latter situation the patient is suddenly wakened gasping for breath and the only way relief can be obtained is by assuming an upright position.

When a diuretic is ordered, accurate recording of fluid intake and output is important. Recording of blood pressure may be necessary as it is often raised in this condition. As digoxin may be used for its stimulant effect on cardiac muscle, pulse rate should be recorded frequently and any change in rhythm reported.

The patient will be confined to bed, so good basic nursing care is essential, with attention to pressure areas, oral hygiene, bed bathing, encouragement with diet, and assistance with feeding when necessary as he will feel weak and be easily exhausted. Mobilisation will require to be started slowly, a little more time being spent out of bed each day.

Another problem which can arise is constipation, especially in the early stages of the illness, probably due to the patient's inability to use a bedpan without giving rise to great respiratory distress and as a result he will not make the extra effort of defaecation. To prevent this giving a small daily dose of senakot syrup or liquid paraffin emulsion will be of benefit and encourage effortless emptying of the rectum.

The patient may sometimes be allowed out of bed to use the commode.

Nursing Care in Myocardial Infarction

On admission the patient is often acutely ill, frightened and agitated. Reassurance is essential and one must gain the patient's confidence and co-operation.

In appearance he will frequently look ill, being pale, perspiring profusely, clinically shocked, and possibly dyspnoeic and cyanosed. Chest pain may be severe, resembling a crushing band around chest, and it may radiate across the left side of chest, upwards to the throat and neck and down the left arm. Chest pain can be very slight amounting to only a feeling of discomfort but this does not mean that the patient is any less ill.

The most important issues are, the relief of pain, and making the patient comfortable with as little movement as possible.

If the patient comes into the ward fully clothed, the bed can be easily covered by placing a sheet or special blanket over the base, and he may then lie on this until he can be undressed after the pain has been relieved.

Undressing can be done with very little upset to the patient, but again one must explain what is to be done so that he may co-operate. Once he has been undressed position in bed is important. It is usually found that two pillows under the head give enough support and encourage relaxation. There are, however, very few patients who enjoy being fed, therefore for mealtimes only the patient may be comfortably supported by three pillows. There are times when a patient is too ill to wish food but will take fluids, which he must have at regular intervals and with which he must be given every assistance. To do this the patient's head should be supported by the nurse placing her hand beneath the pillow. He may wish to hold the cup himself, if not, holding the cup steadily and giving the drink slowly will prevent him choking.

If the patient is dyspnoeic on admission, he will be more comfortable propped up with several pillows. A bedcage is essential to allow free movement of the lower limbs, which should be encouraged to prevent the possible development of a deep vein thrombosis.

Pulse rate, rhythm and volume should be recorded regularly. If the patient is hypotensive the physician will probably wish the blood pressure to be recorded at frequent intervals.

Drug therapy will depend on the patient's needs and will be prescribed by the physician.

Good general nursing care is essential, with particular attention to pressure areas, oral hygiene and toilet care. As has already been mentioned leg movements are important, these may be passive at first — done by the nurse or physiotherapist.

The patient may remain in bed for one to six weeks, depending on the wishes of the physician in charge. When he is ready for mobilisation this should be started slowly – on the first day, sitting out of bed for ½ hour, on the second day, 1 hour, and possibly on the fourth day, a short walk may be taken, thereafter increasing the amount done each day until full mobilisation is attained probably by the end of one week.

Nursing Care in Deep Vein Thrombosis

Special points on nursing care:–

1. Elevation of the foot of the bed to relieve tension due to oedema which develops as a result of thrombosis. A bedcage is necessary to prevent pressure by the bedclothes on the limbs.
2. The physician will advise as to when the patient may commence leg exercises and the physiotherapist will be of help in instructing the patient in exercises which will be of greatest benefit after the acute phase.
3. When the patient is allowed out of bed to sit on a chair it is important to keep the affected limb elevated and full mobilisation will no doubt be encouraged by the physician as soon as possible.
4. The treatment prescribed is usually the administration of anti-coagulant drugs, intravenously and orally, the regime chosen will be decided by the physician in charge. When the patient is on anti-coagulant therapy one must always be alert for any signs of internal bleeding, e.g. by testing stools and urine daily for blood, and a positive result must be reported immediately.

The patient will usually be on anti-coagulant therapy for some time after discharge from hospital and it is therefore important that he understands the action of the drug and what precautions to take in the event of injury or other treatment. Patients are often given a card to carry around at all times stating drug and dose.

5. Supply of elastic stockings to give support to the affected leg.

While the patient is in bed frequent attention to pressure areas is very important. The patient is not able to move in bed very easily due to the pain and swelling of the affected leg. Pressure on the heels and buttocks is therefore very constant and the patient should be assisted in changing position every hour.

Nursing Care in Pulmonary Embolism

This is often a complication of deep vein thrombosis. A small clot of blood breaks off and travels to the right side of the heart, from there it passes to the pulmonary circulation and lodges in one of the pulmonary vessels. When this occurs the patient often experiences acute chest pain and dyspnoea, the pain being increased by inspiration and he tends to try to reduce pain by taking shallow breaths.

Treatment will follow probably the same lines as for deep venous thrombosis. The patient will, however, need great encouragement during the acute stage because of the severe pain which tends to discourage movement.

Nursing care is as for all patients on partial or complete bed rest.

Nursing Care of the Hypertensive Patient

Medical treatment is of most importance in this condition, but it is the nurse's duty to report any changes she may observe in the patient during his treatment.

What are the other duties of a nurse in this situation?

> Firstly, to make the patient feel relaxed and confident, so ensuring co-operation during treatment.
>
> Secondly, but no less important, to make sure that the patient takes the treatment prescribed.

Diet may also be of importance to the patient's progress.

While on treatment, the patient will be advised against changing position suddenly as this may cause light headedness or even loss of consciousness.

Recording blood pressure at specified times, should be done while the patient is at rest and again when standing at the bedside, the latter being a useful criterion for the assessment of drug control. Pressure readings can be very satisfactory while the patient is at rest but may drop dramatically when he stands out of bed. It is therefore important to encourage him to be as mobile as possible in the ward.

The patient may experience difficulty with vision, weakness and even loss of consciousness during a hypotensive attack; these can be very alarming. The most important step to be taken, is either to put the patient back to bed and keep him flat until he recovers, or if he collapses on to the floor it is advisable to leave him lying there until recovery, which is usually rapid, occurs.

Nursing Care of a Patient Following Cerebro-Vascular Accident

The patient may be conscious or unconscious, and there may be total loss of power on one side or only slight limb weakness. If the patient has loss of power on the right side there may be loss of ability to speak or difficulty with speaking.

Incontinence of urine and faeces may be present and if the patient is conscious this can cause great distress. There may be occasions when there is retention of urine with overflow incontinence and one must always have this in mind.

When the patient becomes aware of his disability, it gives rise to much mental anguish, he feels quite helpless and although medical and nursing care are important, these will be of little help if he has not the will to improve. One of the first things a nurse must do, is to give her patient encouragement and the wish to try a little more each day.

The Unconscious Patient

The most important point is to keep the airway clear. Much the best way of doing this, is to keep the patient well round on his side with a pillow supporting the back. This is especially important if the patient is vomiting. Frequent change of position is essential, being performed at one or two hourly intervals, depending on the patient's general condition. Oral hygiene should receive attention each time the patient is turned.

Some patients tend to collect mucus in the pharynx and it may be necessary to suck this out using a whistle tip catheter and gentle suction.

Frequent observation of the patient is important in order to assess any change in his condition. Bladder catheterisation may be advised, and although an indwelling catheter can be a source of infection, this can usually be more easily treated than can a pressure sore caused by the patient lying on a wet drawsheet.

The Conscious Patient

This patient requires very active care, and as has already been mentioned continuous encouragement is essential. Early mobilisation and physiotherapy are both important, as they give the patient hope. Physiotherapy is vital, not only to develop and improve muscle tone on the affected side, but to encourage the unaffected side to develop and compensate for the loss of power. Necessary too, will be exercises to encourage co-ordination of movement.

Mobilisation is not the only aspect of care which is important, as the patient's greatest wish is to be independent. Nurses are often guilty of forgetting that patients do not want to be dependent all the time. They will accept help at first, but determination and ingenuity can master many of the difficulties to be overcome. Feeding can be made easier if the food is cut up prior to serving, it can be kept hot by using a plate manufactured by a company producing baby food — the base of which can be filled with hot water, the plate section is fixed over this and the whole plate is firmly held in position on the tray by suction and by the use of modified cutlery.

Modified Cutlery

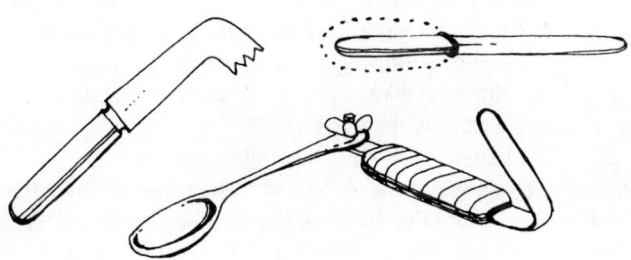

Although the patient will be bedbathed, washing of face and hands will still be necessary at some other points during the day, and the patient will find that by using a foam sponge he can manage to complete this task with very little assistance.

There is one final point to be stressed concerning the patient who has loss of or difficulty with speech, one must always remember that he can hear and understand although unable to answer.

Nursing Care in Diabetes Mellitus

Points to remember concerning general management of a diabetic patient admitted to the ward.

1 *Insulin*

Giving the correct dose of the type of insulin ordered

2 *Diet*

Adequate in carbohydrate allowance and calorie value to meet the patient's daily requirements.

3 *Urinalysis*

Specimens to be tested for sugar and acetone before main meals and before settling at night.

The above applies when the admission is routine and one wishes to cause as little upset as possible to the diabetic control.

However, when a diabetic is admitted as an emergency the situation is entirely different.

There are three reasons for admitting a diabetic as an emergency:—

1. The undiagnosed diabetic — often a young, acutely ill person, thin, dehydrated and often comatose. The relatives may give a history of the patient's increasing thirst and polyuria over a brief period prior to his admission.
2. The patient is a known diabetic and is in a state of diabetic (hyperglyaemic) ketosis.
3. The patient is in hypoglycaemic coma.

The nurse can do very little on her own when the patient is first admitted, except ensure that he is comfortably settled in bed. After she has done this she can, with her knowledge of the probable form of treatment, make suitable preparations.

For 1 and 2 — The Undiagnosed Diabetic and the Patient in a State of Diabetic Ketosis

a Prepare for administration of intravenous fluids. For this one will require a trolley with

1 on the lower shelf —

sterile swabs	crepe bandage
cotton wool balls	micropore or adhesive tape
drapes and a gallipot	a selection of intravenous cannulae
skin cleansing agent	an infusion set
splint	

2   The top of the trolley should be clean and ready to
receive the sterile articles as required. The infusion set
must be primed and ready for connecting to the
intravenous cannula — it is most important to have
the tubing of the infusion set free of air bubbles.

Great difficulty may arise with venepuncture due to the veins collapsing whenever the needle is inserted and venesection (which is a minor surgical procedure to expose one of the veins) may be necessary, one should always have a pack containing the necessary instruments for this procedure on the trolley.

   b   Have ready soluble insulin, syringes and needles.

   c   As there will, in all probability be an electrolyte imbalance, sterile Sodium Bicarbonate and Potassium Chloride should also be available for the physician to use.

   d   Bladder catheterisation is usually advised in order to follow output and to obtain a specimen of urine at frequent intervals for urinalysis.

   e   Once the acute phase is under control the physician will give instructions as to the regime he wishes the patient to have, in the way of intravenous fluids and soluble insulin.

As soon as possible (following these initial steps) the patient should be encouraged to take oral fluids and with further improvement a calorie controlled diet. At first he will be given soluble insulin by sliding scale the dose being regulated by urinalysis. This will eventually be changed when the total daily requirement of insulin can be assessed and one of the prolonged acting insulins can be used as replacement in order to give the patient only one dose of insulin each day.

By the time the patient is ready to leave hospital, insulin dose and dietary requirements will be stabilised.

With the previously undiagnosed diabetic, there are other problems to be overcome before he leaves hospital. Firstly, the patient's own reaction when told by the physician of his illness. At the beginning he will no doubt, appear to understand and accept the full meaning of the condition but after a while there is sudden realisation of all the implications involved in having to take a daily injection of insulin and keeping to a diet, and it is at this stage that the nurse is turned to for answers and reassurances. In order to make the patient feel confident to cope with the situation, one must sound confident in one's answers, and ask the physician to speak with the patient again. The important point to stress is the element of normality, that work, sport and hobbies, do not require to be stopped or changed because of the disease. Attention can be drawn to the excellent Associations which are formed to help Diabetics.

Before the patient is discharged, he must be able to draw up and give his own insulin, or if he is too young his parents must understand how to do this. He must be able to test his own urine and understand his diet. The patient must also realise the importance of keeping to a specific diet and if possible the dietician should be given the opportunity of speaking with the patient and his parents before discharge from hospital is arranged.

The physician in charge of the patient may decide that it would be beneficial both to him and to his parents if a hypoglycaemic state is experienced and observed and to know the emergency measures to reverse this situation.

For 3 (Hypoglycaemic Coma)

In this state the patient is drowsy, sweating profusely, has difficulty with vision and is very confused. He requires glucose urgently, either orally or intravenously. If the patient is conscious oral administration in adequate amount may be possible, this can be given in the form of 50 G. glucose dissolved in water or if "Lucozade" is available it may be more easily tolerated by the patient. If the intravenous method is to be used, the physician will require one or more ampoules of 50 ml. of 50% dextrose solution a syringe and a needle.

As in any acute illness while the patient is in bed, good general nursing care is essential. This includes attention to pressure areas, oral hygiene and toilet care. In some cases it may be necessary to record temperature, pulse and respiration rate at four hourly intervals. Blood pressure may also require to be recorded frequently. Urinalysis is done at specified times, usually before meals, but in the acutely ill patient, more frequently. It is also important that fluid balance charts are accurately maintained.

If a diabetic patient is admitted to the ward for investigation of some other condition, there may be occasions when alteration in diet and time of giving insulin is necessary, in preparation for tests or X-rays, especially if he requires to be fasted overnight. In these circumstances one must be guided by the physician in charge of the patient's treatment.

Giving Insulin

Insulin is usually given by subcutaneous injection, but during the acute phase in Diabetic Ketosis, the injection will be given intramuscularly or intravenously, the latter, of course, being done by the physician.

Insulin is available in three strengths and there are many types each with different properties. When giving insulin one must be very careful — this point cannot be overstressed — to give the correct dose of the correct type ordered.

The strength of insulin available is either, 20 units/ml., 40 units/ml., or 80 units/ml. The aim is to give the patient as small an injection as is possible and this is where the greater strength of insulin comes into use, e.g. for 48 units — a large injection if using 20 strength insulin. In this instance either 40 strength or 80 strength insulin can be used. The dose would be, using 40 strength — 24 marks on the syringe. Using 80 strength — 12 marks on the syringe.

To calculate the correct dose using the greater strength can be confusing and it is important you understand how the above answers are achieved.

40 Strength

Twice as many units/ml. therefore half as many marks are required in the syringe to give the correct dose.

80 Strength

Four times as many units/ml. therefore quarter of the number of marks are required in the syringe, to give the correct dose.

Always have insulin checked as to the correct type being given and the correct dose being drawn up. Always use an insulin syringe as they are specially marked for the purpose.

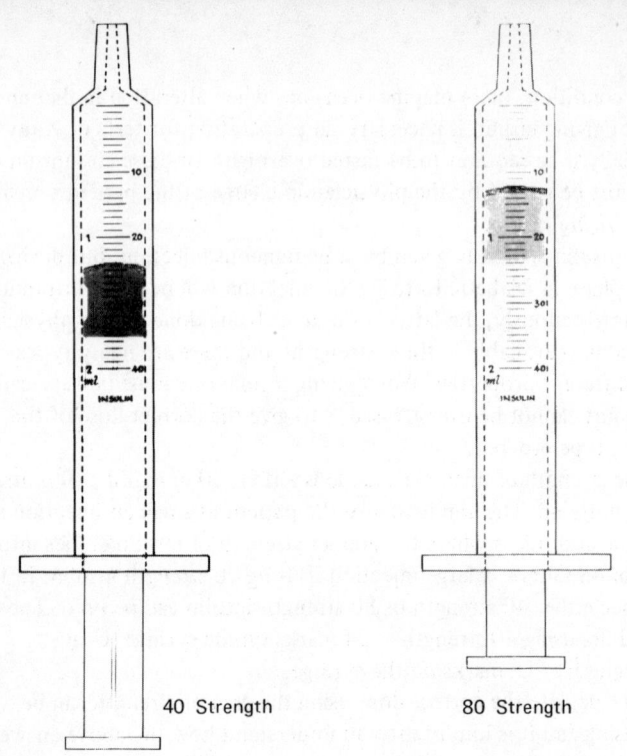

The same 'dose' of insulin showing the quantities in different strengths.

The sliding scale of insulin is a scale set by the physician to control the amount of insulin given to a patient usually during the acute phase of diabetic ketosis. The dose to be given depends on urinalysis e.g. e.g. orange – 30 units; yellow – 20 units; green – 10 units; blue – nil – and may be given four hourly; but this is only an example and must not be accepted as the only scale that can be used. When using a sliding scale *soluble* insulin only is used.

Nursing Care in Thyrotoxicosis

On admission the patient will often be agitated and anxious, and have a rapid pulse frequently due to atrial fibrillation. He should therefore be encouraged to rest as much as possible while in the ward for treatment. The most important point in nursing management concerns drug therapy. If the patient has been given antithyroid drugs given to reduce activity of the thyroid gland and he complains of, for instance, a sore throat, this should not be ignored. It should be reported at once to the medical staff as these drugs can give rise to agranulocytosis. Such drugs, however, may not inhibit thyroid action as hoped and surgery or giving the patient a measured dose of radio active iodine may be necessary. In preparation for the former the patient will be given a course of Lugols Iodine or Potassium Iodide.

While he is in the ward and on drug therapy the physician may request recording of the "sleeping pulse", as this is of value in assessing the patient's progress. The pulse rate is recorded usually between 2 a.m. and 3 a.m. and should be done without disturbing the patient from sleep.

Nursing Care for the Patient with Jaundice

Medical treatment will depend on the underlying cause, but the nurse should report on the colour of the patient's stools and urine, and the amount of vomitting and type of vomitus. Any changes in the patient's colour should be noted. Encourage him to have an adequate fluid intake. It is very probable that he will be disinclined to eat but if not a very light diet is usually most easily tolerated.

Some patients will be confined to bed and in this instance good general nursing care is again important. Daily bathing can give the patient considerable comfort as often accompanying jaundice there is irritation of the skin. Applications of dusting powder frequently will assist in keeping the skin cool.

Nursing Care for the Patient with Respiratory Infection

Although these conditions are all different and require different treatment the nursing care is usually very similar.

The patient will be pyrexial; disinclined for diet; lethargic; and feel generally ill. With antibiotic therapy improvement is usually fairly rapid. Nevertheless good general nursing care is essential with attention to pressure areas at frequent intervals, oral hygiene, encouragement with fluids and diet. Tepid sponging to bring down temperature and to make the patient more comfortable is desirable. There may be occasions when oxygen therapy will be necessary but it cannot be over stressed that there is a danger in giving oxygen without first getting the physician's advice as to the rate of flow and type of mask to be used. There are many patients, especially the middle aged and elderly, who have chronic respiratory problems, to whom a high rate of flow of oxygen would be disastrous as the carbon dioxide level would rise within the blood causing toxicity and death.

Physiotherapy is of great assistance to the patient, exercises to encourage deep breathing and therefore causing improved ventilation of lung tissue with loosening of the secretions which gather as result of inflammatory changes, assistance with coughing to rid the bronchial tubes of the excess secretions and encourage expectoration. It is important that specimens of sputum are obtained and sent to the laboratory for examination.

Nursing Care for Patients with Anaemia

There are several different types of anaemia and many conditions which can cause it. All patients admitted with anaemia for investigation will require nursing management according to their severity, some may be confined to bed, others fully ambulant, each requiring quite different levels of intensity of nursing care.

Investigations are of great importance and the nurse has a vital role to play in these if accurate results are to be obtained. The tests performed will depend on the suspected cause and may include sternal marrow puncture or iliac crest biopsy and histamine test meal, all of which are described under "Special Diagnostic Procedures." Stools and vomitus, if any, should be tested for occult blood which may be present if there is bleeding from any point within the gastro-intestinal tract e.g. from a duodenal ulcer. Faecal collection over a period of four or five days may be required for testing at laboratory level for evidence of malabsorption. Another aspect of importance is the patient's diet prior to admission, since it is all too common for a young busy mother to feed the family and forget about herself or an elderly person to get out of the habit of eating meat or even cooking because of either expense or lack of interest, each giving rise to possible iron deficiency. On occasions the physician may request the dietician to make a dietary survey of the patient's eating habits prior to admission.

Nursing Care

The very ill or the undernourished debilitated patient will require attention to pressure areas and changing of position in bed very frequently. Oral hygiene and encouraging adequate fluid intake to prevent infection of the mouth is important, as is care of the skin by bathing every day or on alternate days as the patient's condition will allow. Observation of diet intake is necessary as often he feels unable to eat or cannot summon up the energy to make the effort to do so, therefore small nutritious meals are important and assistance may be given with feeding where necessary.

The acutely ill patient will receive treatment as soon as possible, and this could be by blood transfusion. The responsibilities of the nurse in this situation are already mentioned within the text.

Treatment is dependent on the underlying cause of the anaemia and the appropriate therapy will be ordered by the physician when results of investigations are available.

Nursing Care for Patients with Haematemesis and Melaena

Both are the visible evidence of bleeding within the gastro-intestinal tract.

Haematemesis — vomiting of blood, fresh or altered.

Melaena — presence of blood in faeces.

Nursing Care

This will in many respects be influenced by the cause, the condition of the patient and the treatment required.

The emaciated patient, will, of course, require very active care, oral hygiene and pressure areas being of particular importance. Encouragement with diet and fluids if allowed will be necessary. If he is vomiting oral intake will probably be restricted and fluids will be given intravenously. In addition he may have a naso-gastric tube in position which will require to be aspirated at regular intervals. The aspirate must be measured and tested on each occasion for the presence of blood if it is not obvious. The importance of maintaining an accurate fluid balance chart must be stressed especially when active bleeding is apparent and blood replacement necessary. Frequent recording of blood pressure and pulse rate will be necessary during the acute phase. A rise in pulse rate can be significant and must be reported as it is usually an indication of fresh bleeding often before there is visible evidence of this.

The patient may, however, not be an acute admission, but in the ward for investigation of suspected gastro-intestinal blood loss. X-rays are of great importance when a diagnosis has to be made, but they can be of little value if the patient has not had adequate preparation, e.g. of bowel prior to a barium enema. This is the responsibility of the nursing staff and must be done correctly. Other diagnostic procedures may be undertaken at the discretion of the physician in charge.

Treatment will depend on cause and as acute or chronic gastro-intestinal blood loss will cause anaemia this will require correction.

Nursing Care for Patients with Ulcerative Colitis

This is an acute dehydrating and incapacitating illness, caused by inflamation of the colon.

Nursing Care and Observation

Frequent testing of stools for blood and observation of stools for colour and presence of mucus is important. The results should all be charted in order to enable the medical staff to assess the patient's condition. Fluid balance charting is important as there will be considerable fluid loss with diarrhoea. The patient should be encouraged to take light roughage-free meals and adequate fluid intake. In severe cases intravenous fluid replacement will be necessary. Care of the skin around the anal region with application of a Barrier cream after each bowel movement is often desirable.

Frequent attention to all pressure areas is essential. Often the patient is very thin and wasted and will develop pressure sores easily. Attention to oral hygiene and giving mouth washes is also an important duty. Temperature, pulse and blood pressures may require to be recorded four hourly.

Nursing Care of the Epileptic Patient

The patient may be admitted to the ward for two reasons.
1. He may be in Status Epilepticus.
2. He may have had an epileptic seizure prior to admission and is brought into the ward for observation and possible alteration in drug therapy.

Nursing Management

The patient may be conscious or unconscious, in either state he will require constant observation and supervision.

Protection of the patient against possible injury must rate high in the nurse's responsibilities. Cot sides should be fixed to the bed in order to prevent the patient rolling out during a seizure. Pillows may be placed round the patient to prevent him striking himself on any hard surface. Dentures should be removed as they could be broken and inhaled. If the patient has his own teeth there is danger of him biting his tongue during a seizure, therefore, a padded metal spoon or spatula which can be put in the mouth to prevent injury to the tongue, should be conveniently placed at the bedside — NEVER attempt to put ones fingers in the patient's mouth to separate the clenched teeth before inserting the spatula.

Observation is very important in order to report to the physician on frequency and severity of seizures and the time over which a patient has loss of consciousness. When the patient recovers from a seizure he will probably be very drowsy and emotionally upset, therefore he will require reassurance and understanding.

Bed rest will possibly be advised until the seizures are fairly well controlled. When the patient is allowed up, it is still important for the nurse to maintain frequent observation. It may be necessary, initially, to escort him within the ward until a full assessment of the effectiveness of the drug therapy is made.

Nursing Care in Acute Poisoning

In the acute medical ward there is always the possibility of admitting a patient who has by intent or in error taken an overdose of drugs or some other poisonous substance.

Treatment will depend on the substance taken and may include:—

1. *Gastric Lavage*

   Requirements —

Oesophageal Tube	Pail
Portex connection of appropriate size	Mackintosh
Large Jug containing washout fluid	Lubricant
Small jug	Swabs
Conical funnel	Tubing
Clamp	

The patient lies flat in the lateral position, the mackintosh is placed under the patient's head. If the patient is unconscious the procedure will be done by the physician, otherwise the nurse may be responsible for the lavage.

The oesophageal tube is passed orally as described within the text. After the position of the tube is checked

   1 the funnel with its attached tubing is connected to the oesopageal tube using the portex connection
   2 the tubing is clamped
   3 the funnel is filled with the fluid to be used
   4 the clamp is released allowing the fluid to flow slowly into the stomach
   5 After approximately 500 mls the funnel is inverted over the pail to allow this amount to syphon back.

This procedure is repeated several times until the return is clear. Any tablets or debris in the return fluid should be retained for examination.

2. *"Forced"Diuresis*

   The patient is given large amounts of fluid intravenously over a short period of time — some of the bottles will have supplements added e.g. Potassium Chloride. A diuretic is given to stimulate greater urinary output.

   The patient may be conscious or unconscious. The nurse should have two trolleys prepared for his admission.

   1 For administration of intravenous fluids.
   2 For Catheterisation — this may not be necessary if the patient is conscious.

The patient's response to the measures taken to counteract the poison will depend greatly on the length of time which has elapsed since ingestion and commencement of treatment.

On recovering the patient's reactions to the situation can vary considerably. Sometimes specialist help is necessary with further treatment in a specialised unit, to enable the patient to resolve his problems. The patient may however remain in the ward and as a nurse one is inevitably involved in trying to help him. One can give time to the patient but total involvement is not practical as one is depriving other patients of nursing skills. There is in most hospitals a Medical Social Worker who is trained to give the kind of support and help which will be of benefit to the patient.

Section III

Special Diagnostic Procedures

It is often difficult to be able to reassure a patient before any diagnostic procedure, but it is very important that a patient is told beforehand what is going to happen. If the nurse has seen the procedure on previous occasions it is always easier to explain what will take place. Explanations take time, but it is time well spent and usually results in greater co-operation from the patient.

In order to prevent repetition, the trolley used in each of the following procedures, should have as a basic setting

1. sterile swabs
2. cotton wool balls
3. two gallipots
4. drapes

The extra items necessary will be stated.

1. Sternal Marrow Puncture

Requirements:

The basic sterile setting.
masks
one pair sterile gloves
skin cleansing agent
sterile drapes
local anaesthetic
5 ml. syringe
needles for giving local anaesthetic
20 ml. syringe for withdrawing specimen of marrow
sterile sternal marrow needle complete with guard and stilette
nobecutane spray
dressing to apply over puncture area.

In some instances, slides, watch glass and fine toothed forceps if these are not provided by the haematology department.

The most comfortable position for the patient and the most convenient for the physician, is one in which the patient is reclining in bed with two pillows giving support to both head and shoulders. It is probably easier to remove the gown completely exposing the chest, but always remember to keep the patient covered. The skin over the sternum is, where necessary, shaved.

The physician will then —
- clean the skin
- arrange the sterile drapes around the area to be used
- draw up the local anaesthetic
- inject local anaesthetic into the subcutaneous tissue over the chosen site of the puncture
- the injection is then continued into the surrounding tissue
- finally into the periosteum of the sternum.

After a few minutes, the sternal marrow needle, with its guard already fixed on the shaft is inserted.

When the periosteum is reached
- pressure is exerted
- the needle enters the inner layer of the bone
- the stilette is withdrawn
- the 20 ml. syringe is attached to the needle
- suction is then applied
- marrow granules are aspirated into the syringe

When the physician is satisfied he has obtained a suitable specimen the needle will be withdrawn.
- pressure is applied over the site of puncture for a short time
- the area is sprayed with Nobecutane
- a sterile dressing applied.

There are two occasions when the patient will experience pain:—
  (a) with the injection of local anaesthetic
  (b) when the marrow is aspirated.

otherwise there will only be discomfort. There will be some tenderness over the site of puncture for a few hours afterwards and the patient will require reassurance on this point.

Sternal Marrow Needle with Stilette

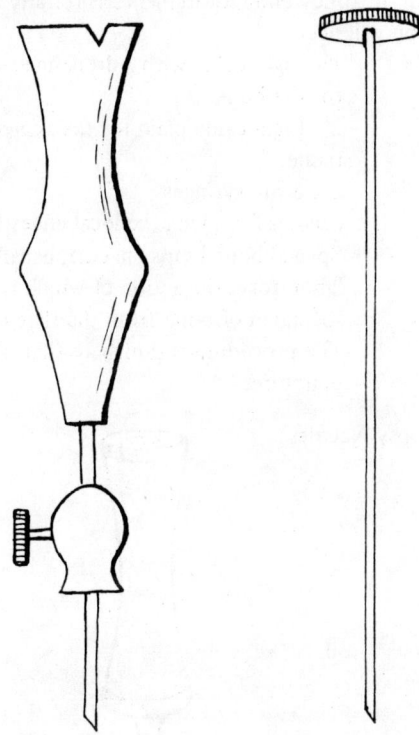

2. Iliac Crest Biopsy

Preparation of trolley and requirements as for any sterile procedure. In addition you will need:—

>1% Lignocaine with Adrenaline as local anaesthetic for the bone.
>
>2% Lignocaine plain for the skin and subcutaneous tissue.
>
>2 x 5 ml. syringes
>
>needles for giving the local anaesthetic
>
>Special bone biopsy needle, usually supplied by the laboratory, the action of which is to punch out the specimen of bone from the Iliac Crest.
>
>The procedure is similar to that of sternal marrow puncture.

Iliac Crest Biopsy Needle

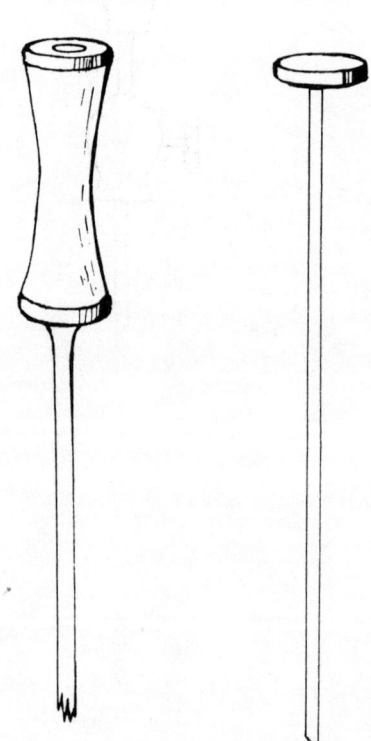

When the specimen is obtained the puncture site must be firmly dressed using swabs and strips of 3 inch elastoplast. The patient should remain on bed rest for at least 24 hours following the procedure and observation of the dressing and area around it should be made frequently as there is a possibility of bleeding and haematoma formation.

3. Fibroscopy

This is a procedure which enables the physician to examine the lining of the stomach without the need for surgery. The instrument used is very specialised, it is a long malleable tube which is illuminated at the tip and lined by small mirrors which reflect the image when the tube is in position in the stomach. It is approximately 2 cm in diameter and is passed over the throat by the physician doing the examination.

Fiberscope

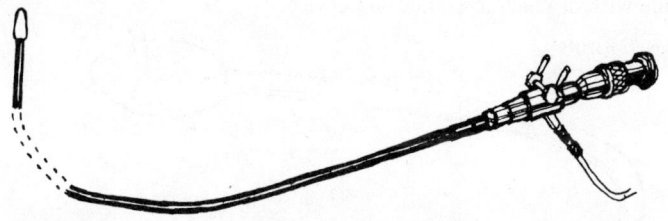

The preliminary preparation is, however, the responsibility of the nursing staff and is important. The patient is fasted overnight, dentures are removed prior to examination, a premedication is ordered and given by injection approximately one hour before examination. As has already been mentioned the fiberscope is passed over the throat, it is therefore essential for the throat to be anaesthetised. Two Benzocaine lozenges to suck — the first 30 minutes, the second 15 minutes before examination, or Lignocaine syrup can be used, but the physician will advise as to the method he wishes used.

To Pass the Fiberscope

The physician will request the patient to lie on his left side, head supported by one pillow, neck fully extended, and held in this position by another member of staff. Once the tube is passed the physician can move it round to enable him to see almost all parts of the wall of the stomach, to make examination easier he can inject air into the stomach by means of a bellows attachment causing the stomach to distend. This can make the patient feel distressed as it will make him belch, otherwise there is very little discomfort while the tube is down.

When the examination is finished the fibrescope is withdrawn, the patient is given a mouth wash and nothing thereafter orally for approximately 4 hours, this prevents accidental inhalation of fluid into the trachea and bronchus as could occur since the throat is anaesthetised.

4. Crosby Capsule

This is a long thin X-ray opaque tube with a Luer fitting at one end to which a syringe can be attached and at the other end a small metal capsule within which is a guillotine device.

Crosby Capsule

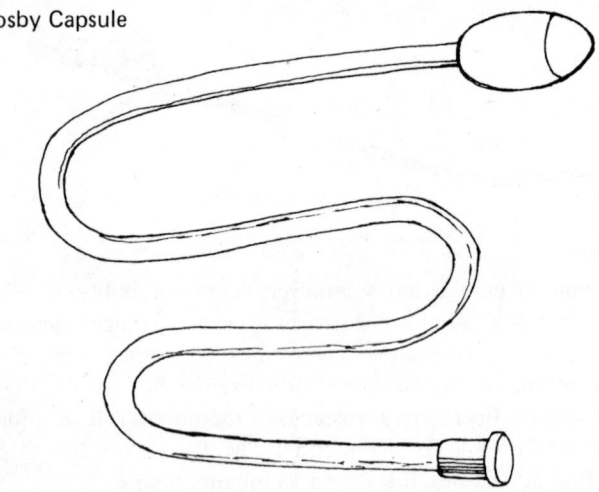

The patient requires to be fasted for this procedure. The capsule is passed by the physician either in the evening and the biopsy taken the next morning or in the morning and the biopsy taken later the same day.

The capsule is placed at the back of the patient's tongue and he is asked to swallow. He should lie on the right side as much as possible as this aids the capsule to move down the gastro-intestinal tract to the level of the jejunum — it is the bowel's normal peristaltic action which carries the capsule into position.

It is very important to ensure that the capsule tubing is firmly fixed at its proximal end. This can be done by tying a tape below the Luer fitting and pinning the ends of the tape to the patient's gown. As a double safety measure this end of the tubing can be securely attached to the side of the patient's face with micropore tape.

Before the biopsy is taken the position of the capsule is checked either by single X-ray or by screening — the latter is more frequently used as the position of the tube can be altered during the screening if necessary.

To take the biopsy

Requirements: 20 ml. glass syringe.

Liquid paraffin to lubricate the piston.

Filter paper on which to put the specimen.

Fine dissecting forceps, scissors.

A container in which there is preservative into which the specimen will be placed.

The physician will attach the syringe to the end of the tube, he will pull the piston up several times to create a vacuum within the tube and cause the lining of the bowel to be pulled into the side of the capsule. The piston is finally drawn up and released sharply, this causes the guillotine device within the capsule to be activated and the specimen obtained. The tube is withdrawn and the specimen of tissue is removed from within the capsule. It is placed in the container with preservative and sent to the laboratory for examination under the microscope.

The patient should be given a mouth wash when the tube is withdrawn. It is important to observe the patient's pulse rate for a few hours after withdrawal of the capsule for evidence of bleeding from the biopsy site. A light roughage free diet is advised for the following 24 hours.

5. Renal Biopsy

Prior to this procedure the patient will have had an intravenous pyelogram and the films must be available for the physician to refer to at the time of the biopsy.

Requirements: The basic sterile pack
renal exploration needle
renal biopsy needle
local anaesthetic
5 ml. Syringe
needles
sterile scalpel blade, gown and gloves
skin cleanser
face masks
strips 3" elastoplast for final dressing.

Renal Biopsy Needle

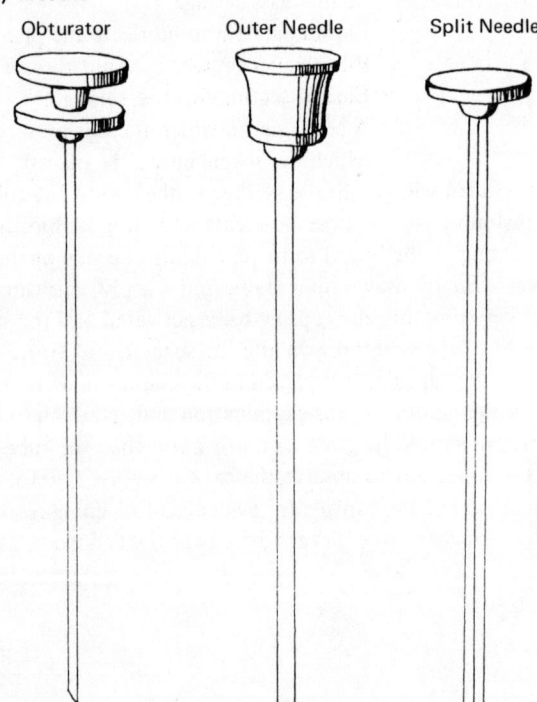

Obturator　　　　Outer Needle　　　　Split Needle

The patient is asked to lie in the prone position and a sand bag is placed under the abdomen. The area of the lumber region is marked by the physician — it is at this point that the pyelogram films are essential, measurements are taken from the films and related to the skin surface giving great accuracy for the insertion of the exploration needle. When the kidney position is confirmed the exploration needle is withdrawn and the biopsy needle is inserted. After the biopsy specimen is obtained a very firm dressing is applied over the puncture site. The patient remains in the prone position for an hour and on bed rest for at least 24 hours after the procedure is completed. It is important to observe the patient closely after the procedure for evidence of bleeding or shock with ½ hourly recording of blood pressure and pulse for 4 hours. Urine output should be charted and each specimen tested for presence of blood. Any change in the patient's condition must be reported to the medical staff immediately, especially if the patient complains of pain in the lumbar region or shoulder, or has any difficulty in passing urine.

6. Liver Biopsy

The greatest danger associated with this procedure is severe bleeding into the liver or abdominal cavity and the patient must be closely observed. Recording of pulse and B.P. ¼ hourly for 2 hours, then 1 hourly for 2 hours, and 2 hourly for the remainder of the 24 hours is essential. Any change must be reported immediately to the medical staff.

Requirements: The basic sterile pack
sterile gown and gloves
biopsy needle
50 ml. Syringe with Luer lock
specimen containers, with preservative
skin cleanser
filter paper
dissecting forceps
scissors
Local anaesthetic
5 ml. Syringe
needles
3 inch elastoplast for dressing

The position of the patient is most important. He should be lying flat and as near the edge of the bed as possible, the head supported by one pillow. The rib cage requires to be extended and it may be necessary for a pillow to be placed under the patient at the level of the lower thoracic spine.

The patient has a very important part to play in the procedure as respiratory movements require to be controlled according to the instructions of the physician. Before the procedure the physician arranges to have blood cross matched for the patient and the results of the prothrombin time available. On completion of the procedure a dressing is applied to the puncture area on the skin and bed rest is maintained for at least 24 hours.

Liver Biopsy Needle

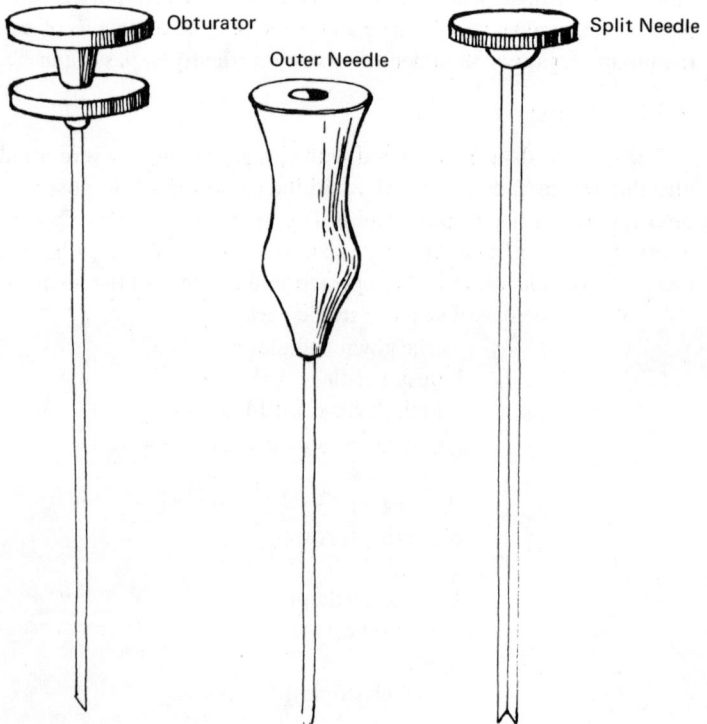

7. Histamine Test Meal

A diagnostic procedure used principally when a patient is suspected of having pernicious anaemia. The purpose of the test is to determine the presence of free hydrochloric acid within the stomach, or if initially absent, whether its secretion can be induced by giving the patient a measured dose of histamine subcutaneously.

Preparation

The patient will require to be fasted overnight. He will require to be weighed. To perform the test, it is necessary to have a trolley on which are the following articles;

> Naso-gastric tube which is opaque to X-ray — this is useful in order to check the position of the tube once passed either by single X-ray or screening
> swabs
> lubricant
> gallipot
> 50 ml. syringe with catheter tip
> spigot
> sickness bowl
> drapes
> disposal bag
> litmus paper or pH. paper

The patient is usually more comfortable if he lies in the semi-recumbant position. The tube is passed over the throat and into the stomach. This is the most difficult part for the patient, but if he is instructed to take deep breaths through his mouth during this manoeuvre, rarely does any difficulty arise. As has already been mentioned it is always advisable to have the position of the tube checked once it has been passed to ensure that it is lying in the body of the stomach — in order to avoid unnecessary delay this can usually be arranged with the X-ray department beforehand.

The gastric contents are now aspirated and put into a container marked "fasting specimen." Before proceeding further, the pH. must be known — this is the level of acidity or alkalinity of the gastric juice. Once the pH. is known, check with the physician as to whether the histamine has to be given — there is the possibility that the test will not proceed further if the pH. reading is under 5 as this indicates the presence of free hydrochloric acid. Before giving histamine the patient must have an injection of an antihistamine drug intramuscularly. Thirty minutes after this injection the patient will be given the injection of histamine *subcutaneously* in a dose calculated according to body weight. Always have the calculations checked and the drug checked when one is drawing it up. Thirty minutes after giving the injection aspirate the gastric contents and put the specimen obtained into a container labelled "Post histamine specimen." The two specimens should be sent to the Biochemistry Department for accurate assessment of pH. and Total Acidity. The test is now complete. Have a mouth wash prepared for the patient. Withdraw the tube and after a mouth wash the patient may have something to eat.

There are variations of this test, some using continuous suction over the various phases and continuing over a longer period of time.

There are two additional points worthy of mention. Firstly regarding the injections the patient receives. The antihistamine tends to make the patient feel a little peculiar — detached from reality and excitable. The histamine causes dilation of the superficial blood vessels and gives the feeling that the skin is going to burst. This can be quite frightening, but if the patient is warned before receiving the injection of how he may feel there will be no problems. Secondly, one must *always* remember to give the antihistamine before histamine.

8. Aspiration of the Peritoneal Cavity — Paracentesis Abdominis

This is a procedure to drain fluid from within the peritoneal cavity.

The procedure is performed by a member of the medical staff but the nurse is responsible for preparing the trolley and also for observing the patient during and after drainage.

> Requirements: the basic sterile pack
> sterile jug for measuring fluid
> trocar and cannula or No. 0 or No. 1 Braunula
> sterile tubing
> drainage bag

a clamp
skin cleansing agent
local anaesthetic
5 ml. Syringe
needles
sterile scalpel blade
nobecutane spray
dressing

Preparation

Preparation of the patient is important. It is essential to have him lying comfortably in bed well supported by pillows and in a position which will allow greatest drainage to occur. If the procedure has to last several hours it is important to give attention to pressure areas at intervals. This can be done safely if precautions are taken to prevent any movement of the cannula during turning of the patient.

Procedure

The abdominal skin over the area chosen is cleansed with Hibitane. Local anaesthetic is injected into the site. After a few moments the trocar and cannula are inserted — in some instances a small incision is made in the skin before the cannula is advanced. Once in position the trocar is removed and the tubing attached to the end of the cannula and the rate of flow into drainage bag is controlled by means of a clamp attached to the tubing. On completion of drainage the cannula is withdrawn, the puncture sealed with Nobecutane and a dressing applied. A binder or many tailed bandage is sometimes used. This is laid under the patient before starting and is pulled firmly round the patient's abdomen as the abdominal girth reduces.

Observations: It is important to watch for:—
(a) Signs of collapse — pallor, sweating, tachycardia.
(b) Evidence of pain or discomfort.
(c) Rate of flow from cannula.
(d) Pulse rate and rhythm should be recorded ½ hourly during the procedure.

Never hesitate to inform the medical staff of any change in the condition of the patient.

9. Aspiration of the Pleural Cavity

Requirements:
- The basic sterile pack
- pleural aspiration needles
- 3-way adaptor
- large syringe
- measure for fluid
- specimen containers
- local anaesthetic
- 5 ml. syringe
- needles
- disposal bag

The procedure is similar to aspiration of the peritoneal cavity.

The most satisfactory position for the physician and the most comfortable for the patient, is for the latter to be sitting upright in bed with a bed table in front of him on which he can lean and gain support. During the procedure and afterwards, it is the nurse's responsibility to observe the patient for evidence of distress such as *increasing* dyspnoea, *rising* pulse rate, pain and collapse. The recording of pulse and respiratory rates ½ hourly for 4 hours is advisable, reporting any changes immediately to the medical staff. Keep the patient well propped up in bed as this helps breathing and makes expectoration easier. Bed rest is usually advised for at least 24 hours after pleural aspiration.

10. Proctoscopy: Sigmoidoscopy: Rectal Biopsy

Procedures used to examine the rectum and sigmoid colon. These are rarely done under anaesthetic and can on occasions cause distress to the patient. It is necessary to have

- sigmoidoscope
- proctoscope
- battery box
- biopsy forceps
- swabs
- drapes

The patient lies on his side with knees flexed and buttocks as near the edge of the bed as possible. The physician will explain to the patient what he is going to do. The sigmoidoscope is lubricated and

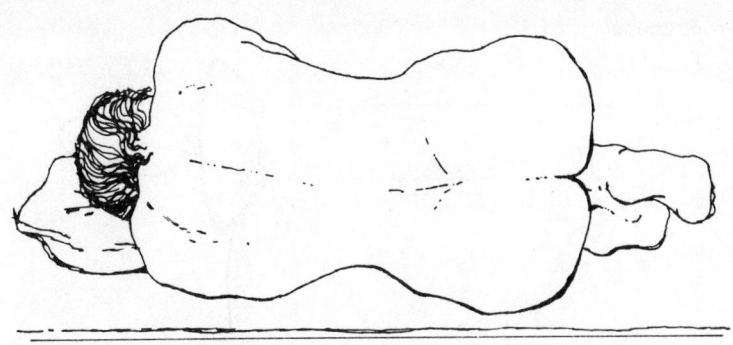

gently passed into the rectum and is advanced as far as possible into the lower colon. The introducer is removed, the light carrier inserted and the electrodes attached to the battery box. When the physician has examined the lining of the bowel he may take a rectal biopsy, the sigmoidoscope is then removed and the patient left in a comfortable position.

Sigmoidoscope

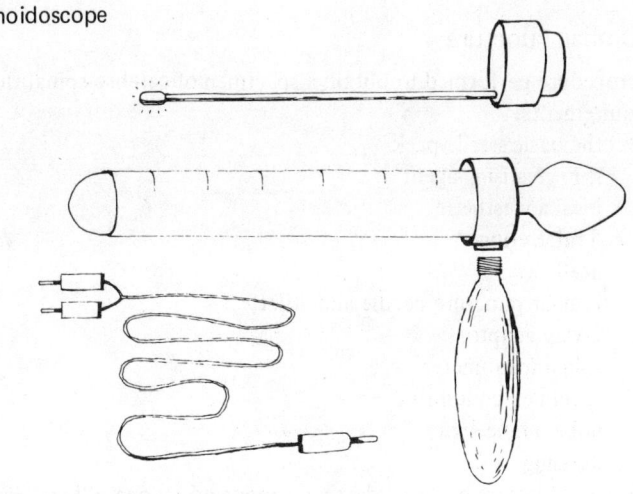

Proctoscope

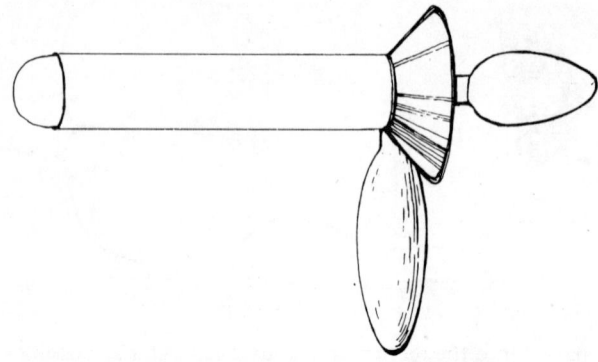

It is the sigmoidoscope which is used when the lower end of the colon is to be examined but the proctoscope when the rectum alone is to be viewed.

If a biopsy has been taken it will be important to observe the patient for evidence of bleeding from the rectum.

11. Lumbar Puncture

A procedure performed to obtain a specimen of cerebro-spinal fluid
Requirements:
> the basic sterile pack
> skin cleansing agent
> local anaesthetic
> 5 ml. Syringe
> needles
> lumbar puncture needle and stilette
> 2-way adaptor
> spinal manometer
> specimen containers
> nobecutane spray
> dressing

The patient lies on his left side head supported by one pillow. His back should be parallel to and as near the edge of the bed as possible.

The patient's hips and knees are flexed, the head is flexed toward the chest. This position causes separation of the vertebrae.

The physician cleans the skin over the area of the 4th and 5th lumbar vertebrae. The local anaesthetic is injected into the skin and subcutaneous tissue. The lumbar puncture needle is inserted, the stilette is withdrawn and the 2-way adaptor is attached. If there is a suspected rise in intra-cranial pressure the manometer will be attached to the adaptor and the pressure checked by allowing cerebro-spinal fluid to flow up into the lumen. Specimens of fluid will be obtained before the needle is withdrawn. When the procedure is completed the puncture site is sprayed with Nobecutane and a dressing applied.

It is important to keep the patient flat for 12 hours following the procedure to prevent him developing headache. He will require routine attention to pressure areas and toilet during this period and assistance will require to be given with feeding.

Manometer
Lumbar Puncture Needle with Stilette 2 Way Adaptor

12. Passing Tubes

The illustrations show the relative positioning of a tube —
Tube Passed Orally

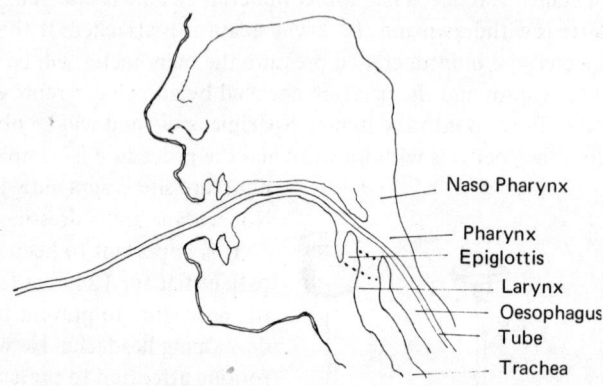

Tube Passed Nasally

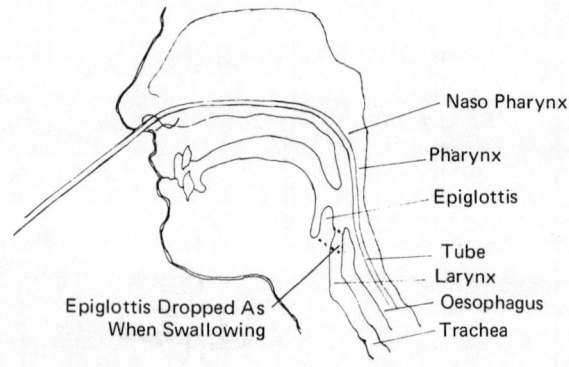

Glossary of Terms

1. Endoscopy — Visualization of the inside of a hollow organ by observation through a tube passed into it e.g. Oesophagoscopy, Sigmoidoscopy.

2. Palliation — Reduction of symptoms of disease without cure.

3. Syndrome — A collection of physical features — symptoms and signs — which commonly occur together.

4. Stricture — A region of narrowing within a hollow organ resulting from disease of its wall.

5. Malaise — A general feeling of lack of well-being.

6. Crepitations — Sounds heard over the lungs and caused by the presence of excess fluid within them.

7. Clubbing — An abnormality of the ends of the digits in which they become inlarged and bulbous.

8. Rigors — Severe involuntary shivering.

9. Angiography — A radiological technique for demonstrating blood vessels by injecting dye into them.

10.	Chromosomes	—	Structures within a cell, on which are carried the genes, which in turn determine the developing characteristics of the cell.
11.	Venesection	—	Removal of venous blood by means of a hollow instrument, needle or catheter, introduced into the vein.
12.	E.S.R.	—	The rate at which red blood cells sediment in whole blood in a standard vertical tube.
13.	Capillaries	—	The smallest blood vessels which transport arterial blood to the veins.
14.	Osteoporosis	—	A degenerative disease of bone in which the supporting structure becomes defective.
15.	Metabolism	—	Relating to the dynamic, energy producing or consuming functions of the body.
16.	Ophthalmoscopy	—	Examination of the inner structures of the eye.
17.	Hypoglycaemia	—	Unusually low level of blood sugar.
18.	Cardiogenic Shock	—	A state of generalised collapse due to heart failure.
19.	Endogenous	—	Arising from within the body.
20.	Pyelography (I.V.P.)	—	A radiological technique for demonstration of the structure of the kidney.

21. Isotope Renography — A technique for assessing renal function involving the administration of radioactive material.

22. Atheroma — Irregular fatty deposits on the inner walls of blood vessels which predispose to thrombosis and occlusion.

23. Hypoxia — A state of oxygen deficiency.

24. Uraemia — Retention of waste products in the blood as a result of renal failure.

25. Electro-Encephalography — (E.E.G.) — recordings of the electrical activities of the brain.

26. Agranulocytosis — Grossly deficient production of white blood cells rendering the patient highly susceptible to infection.

Index

Acromegaly 36
A.C.T.H. 41
Addison's Disease 42
Adrenaline 17, 43
Adrenals 41
Agranulocytosis 99
Alcoholism 12
Allergy 17
Anaemia 25
− Aplastic 28
− Haemolytic 28
− Iron Deficiency 25
− Megaloblastic 26
Antacid 5
Anus 9
Anticoagulent 74
− Drugs 90
Anuria 79
Aortography 59
Arterial Aneurysm 68
Arteriography 63
Arteriosclerotic Disease 69
Ascites 13
Asthma 17
Atheroma 63
Aspiration
− Chest 76
− Peritoneal Cavity 120
− Pleural 122

Bacterial Endocarditis 55
Bacterium Pneumococcus 19
Barium
− Enema 11
− Follow-through 9
− Meal 5
− Swallow 3, 8
Biopsy 115
Bladder Catheterisation 92
Bleeding Disorders 32
Blood 79
− Transfusion 79
− Loss 77

Bone Erosion 34
Bowel
− Large 10
− Small 7
Bronchi 15
Bronchiectasis 18
Bronchiolitis 19
Bronchitis
− Acute 15
− Chronic 15

Cancer 3, 6
Cardiac Catheterisation 55
Cellulitis 63
Cerebral Embolism 55
Cerebro-vascular Accident 69, 92
Cirrhosis 12
Christmas Disease 33
Claudication 44, 63
Clinically Shocked 88
Clinitest 46
Clonic Seizures 65
Coeliac Disease 8
Congestive Cardiac Failure 61
Coronary Artery Disease 56
Creatinine Clearance 83
Crosby Capsule 9
Cushing's Syndrome 41
Cyanosis 86

Deep Venous Thrombosis 62, 90
Diabetes
− Insipidus 37
− Mellitus 44, 94
Diabetic Ketosis 94
Diagnosis 1
Diaphragm 5
Diptheria 69
Disseminated Sclerosis 1, 67
Diuretics 13, 87, 104
Diverticulitis 10
"drip" method of feeding 82
Duodenal Ulcer 7

Duodenum 7
Dyspnoea 79
Dialysis
— Peritoneal 51
Dying—The Care of the 84

E.C.G. 59
Emphysema 15
Empyema 23
Endogenous Creatinine Clearance 59
Enteritis - Regional 9
Epilepsy 65
Epileptic Patient 103
Essential Hypertension 58
Exophthalmos 38
Extradural Haemorrhage 67

'fasting specimen' 119
Fiberscope 113
Fibroscopy 113
Flowmeter 86
Fluids 80
— Loss Of 77
— Balance Chart 75
'forced' diuresis 104
Fundus

Gangrene 44
Gastric Lavage 104
Gastric Ulcer 5
Gastroscope 6
Gout 35
Glomerulonephritis 50
— Acute 48
Gluten 9
Glycosuria 44

Haematemesis 7, 76, 101
Haematoma 113
Haemodialysis 51
Haemolysis 28
Haemophilia 33
Haemoptysis 18
Heartburn 5
Hemiparesis 69
Hepatitis 12
— Infective 11
- Viral 11

Hiatus Hernia 5
High Blood Potassium Levels 51
Histamine Meal 119
Hodgkin's Disease 31
Humidifier 86
Hyperglycaemia 44
Hypertension 44, 58
— Primary 58
— Secondary 58
Hypertensive 69, 91
Hyperthyroidism 38
Hypothyroidism 39
Hypoglycaemia 46, 96
Hypopituitarism 36
Hypotensive 89

Incontinence Of
— Faeces 92
— Urine 92
Infarction of Lung 21
Insulin 44, 94
Intracerebral
— Embolism 68
— Haemorrhage 68
— Thrombosis 68
Intravenous
— Fluids 78
— Pyelography 59, 116
Investigations 1
Isotope Renography 59

Jaundice 12, 99
Jacksonian Epilepsy 65

Kidneys 48

Left Ventricular Failure 60, 88
Leukaemia 29
— Acute 29
— Chronic Lymphatic 30
— Chronic Myeloid 29
Liver 11
— Biopsy 117
Luer Fitting 114
Lumbar Puncture 124
Lungs 19
Malabsorption Syndrome 8, 100
Medical Social Worker 74

Medulla 41
Melaena 7, 25, 76, 101
Menorrhagia 25
Mitral
− Valve 55
− Stenosis 55, 60
Mobilisation 93,
Multiple Myeloma 32
Myocardial
− Infarction 44, 56
− Ischaemia 56, 61

Naso-gastric Tubes
− To pass 82
− Feeding 80
Nephrotic Syndrome 44, 50
Noradrenaline 43

Obstruction 11
Occult Blood 13, 100
Oedema 13, 86
Oesophagoscope 3
Oesophagus 3, 10
Ophthalmoscope 44
Osteoporosis 34
Oxygen 16, 86
− Therapy 100

Palliative 3
Pancreas 44,
Paraesthesiae 69
Parkinsonism 66
Peripheral
− Artery Disease 63
− Neuropathy 44, 69
Peritonitis 11
Pernicious Anaemia 119
Petit Mal 65
Phaeochromocytoma 43
Physical Signs 1
Physiotherapy 20, 93
Pituitary 36
Plasma Cell 32
Pleura 22
Pleural Effusion 19, 23
Pleurisy 23
Pneumococcal 19

Pneumonia 15
− Lobar 19
− Broncho 19
Pneumoconioses 20
Pneumothorax 16, 22
Poisoning 103
Polycythaemia 31
Polydipsia 44
Polyuria 44
Proctoscope 122, 124
Proctoscopy 122
Prognosis 1
Prophylactic 27
Proteinuria 50
Pulmonary
− Angiography 22
− Embolism 21, 91
Pulse Rate 89
Purpura 32
Pyelonephritis 48
Pyloric Stenosis 7

Radiotherapy 3
Reaction to Blood Transfusion 79
Rectal Biopsy 122
Renal
− Biopsy 116
− Failure (acute) 51
− Failure (chronic) 52
− Insufficiency 44
− Transplantation 52
Respiratory Infection 99
Reticulocyte Count 27
Rheumatoid Arthritis 34
Rhythm 89

Scurvy 1
Sigmoidoscope 123
Sigmoidoscopy 122
Shingles 1
'sleeping pulse' 99
Soluble Insulin 98
Spasticity 69
Splenectomy 28
Sputum 15
Status Asthmaticus 17
Status Epilepticus 65, 103

Sternal Marrow Puncture 109
Steroid 9
Stomach 5
Streptococcus 48
Strictures in Bowel 11
Stroke 68
Subarachnoid Haemorrhage 68
Subdural Haemorrhage 67
Sugar 46
– Urine 46
– Blood 46
Symptoms 1

Temporal Lobe Type Epilepsy 65
Thrombocytopenia 32
Thoracotomy 23
Thyroid 38
Thyrotoxicosis 38, 98
Treatment 1
Tuberculosis 23

Ulcerative Colitis 9, 10, 102
Unconscious Patient 85
Urinalysis 94
Urobilinogen 13

Valve
– Stenosed 55
– Incompetent 55
Vascular Accidents 44
Venesection 31
Venography 62
Volume 89
Vomitus 77

Wheezing 17
Whistle-tip Catheter 92

Pages for Notes

The following pages have been left blank intentionally so that as you learn, or researchers discover, you can put a note of it where you will remember where to find it.